D1456664

A Patient's Guide to Glaucoma

Edited by
Young H. Kwon, MD, PhD

Written by:
Young H. Kwon, MD, PhD
John H. Fingert, MD, PhD
Emily C. Greenlee, MD

University of Iowa

Photographs by Ed Heffron, Young H. Kwon, Emily C. Greenlee
Illustrations by Patricia Duffel, John H. Fingert

Published by FEP International Inc.
Copyright 2008

A Patient's Guide to Glaucoma

By Young H. Kwon, MD,PhD; John H. Fingert, MD,PhD; Emily C. Greenlee, MD

Copyright © 2008 by Young H. Kwon, John H. Fingert, Emily C. Greenlee.

Published and distributed by F.E.P. International, Inc.
www.fepint.org
www.medrounds.org/glaucoma-guide

Printed in the United States of America.

For information write F.E.P. International, Inc.
941 25th Avenue #101
Coralville, IA 52241

ISBN   0-9797075-1-X
ISBN13   978-0-9797075-1-3

Advice and suggestions given in this book are not meant to replace professional medical care. The reader is advised to consult his or her physician before undertaking any diet or exercise regimen and in order to gain answers about or treatment for any medical problems. The authors and publisher have made every effort to ensure that drug selection and dosage set forth in this text are in accord with current recommendations and practice at the time of publication. However, because the practice of medicine may change with ongoing research, changes in government regulations, and developments in medicine, the reader is encouraged to read the package insert for each drug for any change in indications and dosage and for added warnings and precautions. This is particularly important when the recommended agent is a new or infrequently employed drug.

MAR - - 2009

About the Authors

Young H. Kwon, MD, PhD, is the Clifford M. and Ruth M. Altermatt Associate Professor of Ophthalmology at the University of Iowa, specializing in glaucoma. He teaches glaucoma to medical students, resident and fellow physicians, and is interested in educating the public about glaucoma. His research interests include glaucoma imaging, cell biology of optic nerve damage in glaucoma, and development of slow-release glaucoma medications.

John H. Fingert, MD, PhD is an Assistant Professor at the University of Iowa specializing in medical glaucoma. His research interests include the molecular genetics and genetic testing for inherited eye diseases.

Emily Greenlee, MD is an Assistant Professor at the University of Iowa specializing in glaucoma and comprehensive ophthalmology. Her primary practice site is at the Veterans Affairs Health Care System in Iowa City, Iowa.

Table of Contents

Chapter 1

Glaucoma: Optic Nerve Disease

1-A. Introduction

The eye is a fascinating organ that allows us to make visual observations about the world around us (Figure 1-1). The complex images we see are transmitted to the brain for processing by way of the optic nerve. Approximately 1.2 million nerve fibers, or *axons*, make up each human optic nerve. The optic nerve travels from the back surface of each eye and joins together at the optic chiasm. The nerve fibers leave the chiasm to the lateral geniculate body as optic tracts. Finally, visual input is transmitted from the lateral geniculate body and travels as optic radiations to the visual area of the brain called the *occipital lobe*. Thus visual images from the retina (the "film" of the eye) travel through the optic nerve, optic tract, lateral geniculate body and eventually to the occipital lobe where the images are processed and interpreted by the brain. Any disease process that affects the optic nerve could disrupt this pathway, leading to visual loss.

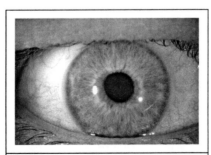

Figure 1-1. The eye

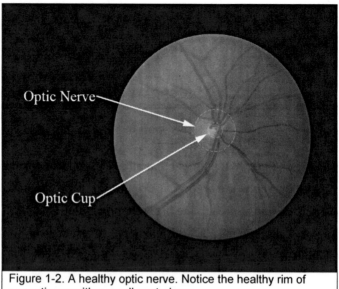

Figure 1-2. A healthy optic nerve. Notice the healthy rim of nerve tissue with a small central cup.

The optic nerve can be damaged by a number of disease entities. Optic neuropathy is a general term used for any condition that damages the optic nerve. Optic neuropathies may be caused by vascular (blood flow) problems, inflammation/infections, metabolic disorders, trauma, tumors, or hereditary diseases. In each case, the result of the disease process is visual loss, which can affect central and/or peripheral vision. Each type of optic neuropathy has characteristic signs and symptoms of visual loss. Some visual losses are temporary, while others are permanent. Some lead to loss of central vision, while others lead to loss of peripheral vision. Those that affect the central vision are more noticeable by patients.

Ophthalmologists (M.D.s specializing in medical and surgical care of the eye) are trained in differentiating various optic neuropathies based on signs and symptoms. Glaucoma specialists are ophthalmologists with additional training in the diagnosis and treatment of glaucoma.

Glaucoma is one type of optic neuropathy. It is a disease of the optic nerve, often (but not always) associated with high intraocular pressure (IOP) resulting from poor drainage of fluid from the eye. There are various types of glaucoma; all share the common feature of optic nerve damage leading to irreversible vision loss. Glaucoma differs from other optic neuropathies by few key features. The main distinguishing feature of glaucoma is "cupping of the optic nerve," which describes the appearance of the optic nerve when it is damaged by glaucoma. While normal optic nerves have a relatively small cup, (Figure 1-2) the optic nerve cup gets progressively larger in glaucoma. Another distinguishing feature of glaucoma is that the treatment is aimed at lowering the intraocular pressure (IOP). The eye has a certain pressure determined by the production and drainage of fluid (called *aqueous humor*) within the eye. The eye fluid is continuously produced and drained from the eye. In patients with glaucoma, normal drainage is impaired, often leading to elevation of IOP.

1-B. The Meaning of Cupping

The term "cupping" of the optic nerve describes the appearance of the optic nerve to the examining eye doctor. When the nerve is viewed through the pupil, it looks like a cup seen from above. The cup is really an empty space in the middle of the optic nerve surrounded by optic nerve fibers. A healthy optic nerve has many nerve fibers traveling through it (approximately 1.2 million fibers), and hence it generally has a small cup. With the loss of nerve fibers from glaucoma, the cup becomes progressively larger because there is less space occupied by the remaining nerve fibers. A clinician can quantify the amount of optic nerve cupping by estimating the cup-to-disc ratio, which can range from 0 to 1 (figure 1-3). The larger the cup-to-disc ratio, the more the optic nerve damage from glaucoma.

3

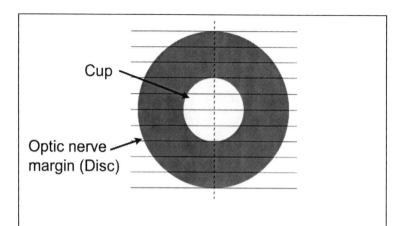

Figure 1-3. The optic nerve is divided into tenths and the cup is compared to the entire optic nerve (optic disc) to obtain the cup-to-disc ratio. The vertical cup-to-disc ratio (along the dotted line) here is 4/10 or 0.4.

In glaucoma the position of the blood vessels within the optic nerve can shift with the progressive cupping, and this can be an important clue that the glaucoma is continuing to cause optic nerve damage. Other exam findings suggestive of glaucoma include hemorrhages (bleeding) on or near the optic nerve. This is commonly seen in poorly controlled glaucoma and is indicative of ongoing optic nerve damage or unstable glaucoma. Glaucoma often affects one eye greater than the fellow eye. If so, there may be asymmetry of the optic nerve cupping between the two eyes. The less affected optic nerve will look less cupped while the more affected eye will look more cupped. Asymmetry of the optic nerves is another clue that can aid in the diagnosis of glaucoma (Figure 1-4).

4

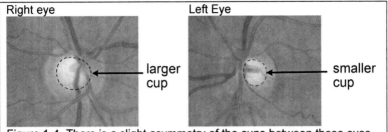

Figure 1-4. There is a slight asymmetry of the cups between these eyes. The right eye (left picture) has a slightly larger cup than the left eye (right picture).

In end stage glaucoma, the nerve may be completely cupped, with no nerve fibers left. In this case the vision may be poor. While most patients that receive treatment will not progress to end-stage glaucoma, those that do may eventually become blind.

It is rare that other optic neuropathies result in cupping of the optic nerve. Most of the time, optic nerve cupping is caused by glaucoma, and the amount of vision loss corresponds to the extent of cupping and optic nerve damage.

1-C. Understanding Vision Loss from Glaucoma

Central vision is the fine vision people use to read and recognize faces, while peripheral vision is the side vision that is used for navigating obstacles in the environment and for detecting oncoming vehicles from a side street. The diagnosis of glaucoma is often made *late* in the disease course, because early stages of glaucoma do not usually cause visual symptoms for patients. Patients often fail to notice peripheral vision loss until it has progressed towards the center of vision. Unless the patient happens to be examined by an eye doctor, they could be unaware that they have glaucoma. The only way to be diagnosed with glaucoma in early stages is to be examined by an eye doctor and undergo an eye exam and visual field testing (Figure 1-5) which measures the amount of vision loss from optic nerve damage (Figures 1-6, 1-7, 1-8, 1-9).

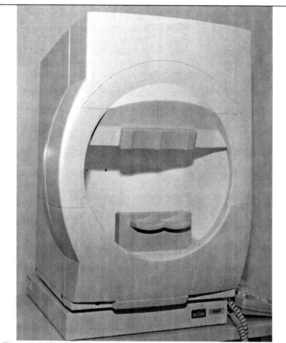

Figure 1-5. Visual field testing with a Humphrey Field Analyzer device (Carl Zeiss Ophthalmic Systems, Inc., Dublin, California) is a standard method for detecting and monitoring glaucoma.

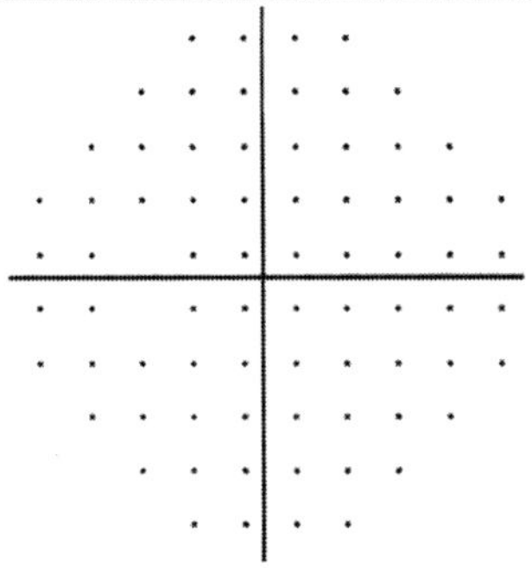

Figure 1-6. Normal Humphrey visual field test. This is a peripheral vision test which is performed to diagnosis glaucoma. There are no dense black spots indicating vision loss.

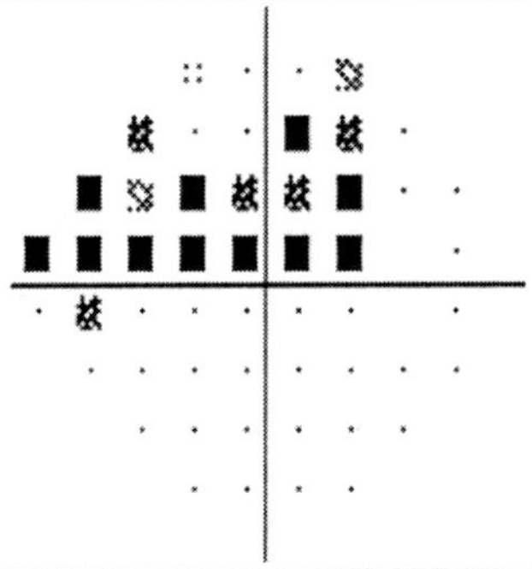

Figure 1-7. Superior visual field loss from glaucoma – as tested by Humphrey visual field device. The black areas represent abnormal blind spots corresponding to areas of vision loss.

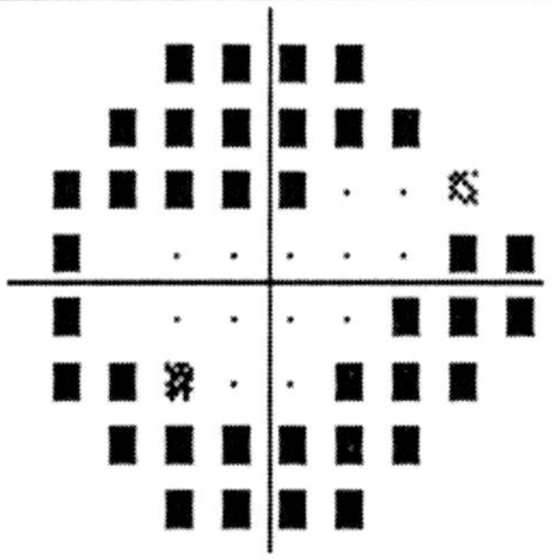

Figure 1-8. Superior and inferior visual field loss from glaucoma causing tunnel vision. Despite the peripheral vision loss, central vision is still intact and the vision may be 20/20.

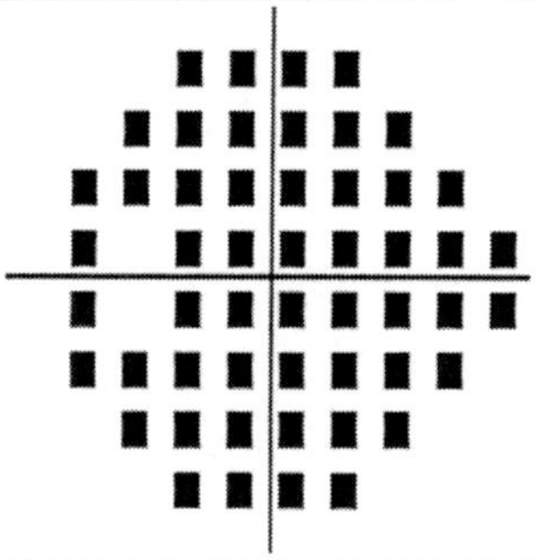

Figure 1-9. End stage glaucoma with dense superior, inferior, and central visual field defects. There is severe visual impairment.

The nerve fibers of the optic nerve enter the nerve head in a well-defined anatomic configuration (Figure 1-10). Glaucoma tends to affect the superior and inferior parts of the optic nerve first, thereby producing arching or *arcuate* visual field defects (Figures 1-7 and 1-8). This explains the characteristic pattern of visual field loss in glaucoma. Because of the anatomy of the eye, when the superior part of the nerve is damaged, patients will develop inferior visual field loss. Conversely, when the inferior nerve is damaged, patients will develop superior visual field loss. Since the center vision is usually spared in the early disease, visual acuity may be 20/20 until later in the disease course. In some patients with glaucoma the central vision can be affected relatively early in the disease process. When the central vision is affected, patients will often notice the vision loss and seek medical help promptly.

If optic nerve damage occurs both superiorly and inferiorly, the two arcuate visual deficits can meet, resulting in tunnel vision (Figure 1-8). Even at this advanced stage of glaucoma, the central vision may be 20/20. However, if the center of the retina is affected (which typically occurs in endstage glaucoma), the central vision will get worse (Figure 1-9). At this point, most of the vision is gone and patients may have difficulty functioning independently.

The visual field test determines the extent of peripheral vision loss. This, in turn, corresponds to the cupping of the optic nerve with glaucoma. Visual field defects from other types of eye diseases may also be detected during visual field testing. Glaucoma has characteristic visual field defects, which correspond to the anatomic distribution of the nerve fibers. Particular patterns of visual field loss can be used to diagnose glaucoma and distinguish it from other eye disorders.

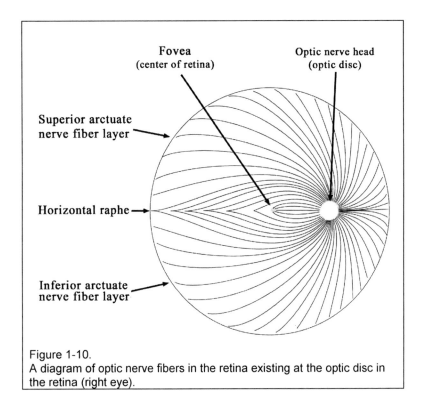

Figure 1-10.
A diagram of optic nerve fibers in the retina existing at the optic disc in the retina (right eye).

1-D. Implications of a Glaucoma Diagnosis

Once a diagnosis of glaucoma is made, there is often fear of blindness and uncertainty about what will happen in the future. Glaucoma is a disease that cannot be cured. However, it can be effectively treated to prevent further vision loss. Patients often fear that they will go blind or that they will have a visual disability. While there are patients who are visually impaired due to glaucoma, this constitutes a minority of patients. If glaucoma is diagnosed and treated early, visual impairment may be minimal or limited.

Once optic nerve tissue is damaged, it is not currently possible to regenerate new optic nerve fibers. The existing visual field defect or decline in vision from glaucoma is permanent. The goal of treatment,

9

therefore, is to preserve the existing optic nerve function. Lowering the eye pressure prevents further optic nerve damage. This is done with eye drops, laser treatments, or surgery.

The importance of regular examination schedule with an eye doctor knowledgeable in the treatment of glaucoma is a key factor in preserving sight in glaucoma. Not only is continuous and periodic monitoring important, but also adherence to prescribed medical or surgical treatment is critical in preserving the sight. Careful adherence to a schedule for taking glaucoma medications and other treatment regimens is often in the hands of the patient (or patient's caretaker) and is the key to treatment success.

Chapter 2

Epidemiology of Glaucoma

2-A. Introduction

Glaucoma represents a significant public health problem. Glaucoma affects more than 67 million people in the world, and approximately 10% of them are estimated to be blind from glaucoma. It is the leading cause of irreversible blindness in the world. In the United States, glaucoma affects more than 2.2 million people, and is the second leading cause of blindness in adults over the age of 40 (the first is macular degeneration).

Glaucoma is not a single disease. There are different types of glaucoma. Glaucoma can be broadly divided into two categories depending on whether or not the drainage angle (called *trabecular meshwork*) in the front of the eye (called *anterior chamber*) is open. The angle is formed at the junction of the cornea and iris. The trabecular meshwork is where the eye fluid (called *aqueous humor*) normally drains out of the eye. If the drainage angle is open on examination, the patient is said to have *open-angle glaucoma*. If the drainage angle is closed on examination, the patient is said to have *angle-closure glaucoma*. Refer to the next chapter (Chapter 3) for detailed description of the eye anatomy, as it relates to glaucoma.

Epidemiology (study of disease in populations) of open-angle glaucoma is sufficiently different from angle-closure glaucoma that each warrants a separate discussion.

2-B. Epidemiology of Primary Open-Angle Glaucoma

The word "primary" of *primary open-angle glaucoma* indicates that no specific cause for the disease has been found to date. Primary open-angle glaucoma (POAG) is associated with optic nerve damage with resultant visual loss. However, POAG may or may not be associated with elevated intraocular pressure (IOP). The normal IOP is between 10 and 21 (in millimeters of Mercury or mm Hg). Classically, POAG occurs in a patient with elevated IOP (greater than 21). However, a significant portion of POAG patients do not have elevated IOP; this subgroup of patients is often referred to as having *normal tension, normal pressure*, or *low tension* glaucoma.

It is estimated that normal pressure glaucoma makes up anywhere from 40-75% of all primary open-angle glaucoma. And POAG makes up 85-90% of *all* glaucomas in the Western world. Prevalence of primary open-angle glaucoma has been extensively studied by a number of well-designed clinical studies in different populations. In white populations, primary open-angle glaucoma is present in 0.3 to 4.0% of the older population (Table 2-1). In Asian populations, POAG is present in 0.5 to 2.6% of the older population. In the Hispanic population in the United States, POAG is present in 2.0%; however, the number of studies on Hispanic populations is limited. In black populations, the prevalence of POAG is higher and ranges from 2.9 to 8.8% of the older population. It is clear that the black population is at a higher risk of developing POAG than in other populations.

Table 2-1. Prevalence of primary open-angle glaucoma in different world populations.	
Race / Location	Prevalence of Primary Open-Angle Glaucoma in older age population . (Generally over age 40)
White populations (US, Europe, Iceland, Australia)	0.3 – 4.0 %
Asian populations (Japan, Mongolia, Singapore, India)	0.5 – 2.6 %
Hispanic population (US)	2.0 %
Black populations (US, Caribbean, Africa)	2.9 – 8.8 %

The risk of developing glaucoma is very small in the general population (see Table 2-1). However, there are several risk factors that are associated with the development of POAG. As seen in Table 2-1, the black race is one such risk factor. Other risk factors include older age, positive family history of glaucoma, elevated intraocular pressure, and thin cornea. A black person has 4 times the risk of developing glaucoma than a white person. The older you are, the more likely you will develop glaucoma. If your first-degree relative (parent or sibling) has glaucoma, your chance of developing glaucoma increases by 2 to 4 fold higher. If your intraocular pressure is over 30 (mm Hg), the chance of developing glaucoma is 40 times greater than if the intraocular pressure is under 15. A thin cornea, which can lead to intraocular pressure measurement error (under-estimation), is also associated with an increased risk of glaucoma. In other words if you have a thin cornea, your true intraocular pressure is higher than what is measured, and you are at a higher risk of developing glaucoma. Additional minor risk factors for glaucoma include myopia (near-sightedness), low diastolic blood pressure, and diabetes, among others. Normal pressure glaucoma has been associated with migraine headaches and *Raynaud's phenomenon* (cold and numb fingers due to poor peripheral blood circulation).

It is uncommon, but possible, for patients to become (*legally*) *blind* from primary open-angle glaucoma. Several studies suggest the risk of becoming blind in one eye for a glaucoma patient can range 15 to 54% over 15 - 22 year period. The risk of becoming blind in both eyes for a glaucoma patient can range from 4 to 22% over the same period. The risk factors for developing blindness from glaucoma include advanced stage of glaucoma at diagnosis, younger age at diagnosis, poor intraocular pressure control, poor compliance with medications, and inadequate treatment and follow-up care. Some of the blindness data are old (from before 1980); with the improvement in treatment over the last 25 years, it is generally believed that the rate of blindness from glaucoma in the 21st century is lower than the figures quoted above.

How do we detect glaucoma early so that we can prevent blindness from open-angle glaucoma? There is no a simple answer. Population screening of intraocular pressure to detect glaucoma has not been very successful, because a significant percentage of patients with glaucoma has normal intraocular pressure. On the other hand, examining everyone by an ophthalmologist would be prohibitively costly and time-consuming. The American Academy of Ophthalmology recommends a complete eye examination (that includes glaucoma screening) every 2-4 years between ages 40-64, then every 1-2 years after age 65 (Table 2-2). If you have risk factors for glaucoma, additional examinations are recommended.

14

Table 2-2. Recommended frequency of eye examinations by American Academy of Ophthalmology		
Age group	No glaucoma risk factors	Glaucoma risk factors
20-29	At least once during interval	Every 3-5 years
30-39	At least twice during interval	Every 2-4 years
40-64	Every 2-4 years	Every 2-4 years
65+	Every 1-2 years	Every 1-2 years

2-C. Epidemiology of Primary Angle-closure Glaucoma

Primary angle-closure glaucoma (PACG) is usually associated with elevated intraocular pressure, optic nerve damage, and resultant visual loss. The aqueous fluid drainage angle becomes progressively narrower (usually with age) and eventually, the intraocular pressure increases as a result of a decrease in aqueous fluid drainage.

Epidemiology of PACG is less well studied than that of open-angle glaucoma. However, it is no less important. In fact, PACG may account for 64% of *all* glaucomas in Mongolia, and 50% of *all* glaucomas worldwide. In the white, Hispanic, and black populations, angle-closure glaucoma is present in 0.1 - 0.6% of the older population (Table 2-3). However in Asian populations, angle-closure glaucoma is present in 0.3% (Japan) to 2.7% (Alaska) of the older population.

Table 2-3. Prevalence of angle-closure glaucoma in different world populations

Race / Location	Prevalence of Angle-closure Glaucoma in the older age population (generally over age 40)
White populations (Europe, Australia)	0.1 – 0.6 %
Asian populations (Alaska, Japan, Mongolia, Singapore, India)	0.3 – 2.7 %
Hispanic population (US)	0.1 %
Black populations (Africa)	0.5 – 0.6 %

Blindness can occur in angle-closure glaucoma as well. In fact, the rate of blindness from angle-closure glaucoma may be higher than that of open-angle glaucoma. Blindness in one eye occurs in 10 –50% of Inuit and Chinese patients with angle-closure glaucoma. In East Africa, blindness in both eyes occurs in 21% of angle-closure glaucoma patients.

Because acute angle-closure glaucoma can be prevented with a laser surgery (Figure 2-1. Chapter 9 will cover this in more detail), there is a great interest in population screening for early detection of angle-closure glaucoma. In reality however, screening for angle-closure glaucoma has been difficult. There are several methods for detection of a narrow (or closed) drainage angle (Figure 2-2). Some are simple (for example, oblique flashlight test), while others require special equipment (for example, Van Herick's test utilizing the slit lamp instrument). Unfortunately, none of these methods meet all the criteria for effective mass screening, which requires quick, easy administration by minimally trained personnel at low cost. Studies are under way to look for the most effective methods to screen for and prevent angle-closure glaucoma in high-risk Asian populations. The population screening and preventive treatment of angle-closure glaucoma is particularly important in Asian countries where the prevalence of angle-closure glaucoma is relatively high. Such screening and preventive treatment of angle-closure glaucoma can have a major impact on public health in those populations.

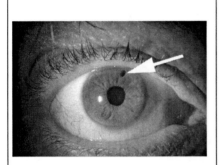

Figure 2-1. Photograph of an eye that has received laser peripheral iridotomy (LPI) to treat acute angle-closure glaucoma. LPI creates a small hole in the iris (arrow) that is visible with an eye examination.

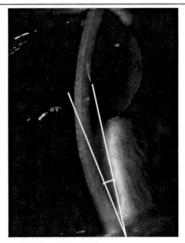

Figure 2-2. Slit lamp picture of an eye in acute angle-closure glaucoma. Notice the drainage angle represented here by 2 intersecting lines is very narrow (about 12°). The angle is also called "irido-corneal" angle because it is formed by the iris and cornea.

Chapter 3

Anatomy of the Eye in Glaucoma

3-A. Normal ocular anatomy

A brief review of the normal anatomy and function of the eye will serve as a basis for understanding the abnormal disease processes that cause glaucoma.

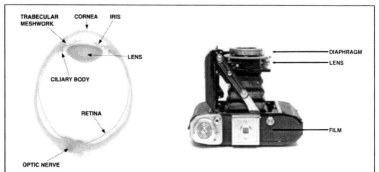

Figure 3-1. Basic anatomy of the eye. Structures of the eye are indicated on the cross-sectional image of a human eye shown on the left and a camera is shown on the right for comparison. (The image of the eye is courtesy of Nasreen Syed, MD, University of Iowa).

Many of the structures of the eye closely resemble the components of a camera (Figure 3-1). The *cornea* and the *lens* focus images on the retina and are similar to the lens of a camera. The *retina* is the tissue of the eye that senses light and functions like the film of a camera. The *iris* controls the amount of the light that enters the eye as the diaphragm regulates the amount of light passing into the camera. Finally, the images detected by the retina are delivered by the optic nerve to the brain where vision is perceived. The *optic nerve* is the part of the eye that is damaged by glaucoma.

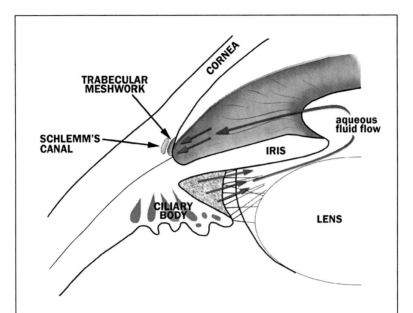

Figure 3-2. Aqueous Fluid Flow in the Eye. The aqueous fluid that fills the eye is produced by the *ciliary body* and flows between the iris and lens, through the pupil and to the drainage angle (junction of the iris and the cornea). Aqueous fluid exits the eye through a tissue called the *trabecular meshwork* in the drainage angle.

3-B. Aqueous fluid production and drainage angle

The cornea and the lens have no blood supply. They receive nourishment from nutrients in the aqueous fluid that fills the eye. The aqueous fluid is produced by the ciliary body, which is located behind the iris (Figure 3-2). The aqueous fluid enters the eye through the ciliary body and flows between the iris and lens through the pupil. The fluid passes out of the eye through a tissue called *the trabecular meshwork*, which is at the *drainage angle* (at the junction of the cornea and the iris). As the aqueous fluid passes through the eye, it supplies the lens and cornea with nutrients and carries away waste products.

19

The pressure of the fluid in the eye (intraocular pressure) is determined by the amount of fluid entering the eye through the ciliary body and exiting the eye through the trabecular meshwork. In most people, the balance between the fluid coming in and going out of the eye results in an eye pressure between 10 and 21 mm of Hg. In patients with glaucoma, there is increased resistance to flow through the trabecular meshwork causing the intraocular pressure to rise.

Eye doctors regularly examine the drainage angle to see if there is any visible obstruction to fluid leaving the eye through the trabecular meshwork. A special lens (*gonioscopy lens*) is needed to examine the trabecular meshwork (Figure 3-3A – 3-3B). The gonioscopy lens is gently placed against the surface of the cornea and allows eye doctors to see the trabecular meshwork in the drainage angle (Figure 3-3C).

There are two major types of glaucoma. In open-angle glaucoma, the drainage angle between the cornea and the iris is open and allows the aqueous fluid of the eye to make its way to the trabecular meshwork – the chief site for fluid drainage from the eye. In patients with open-angle glaucoma, (non-visible) abnormalities in the trabecular meshwork reduce the outflow of aqueous humor. In angle-closure glaucoma the trabecular meshwork is visibly obstructed, and the aqueous humor is prevented from draining out of the eye.

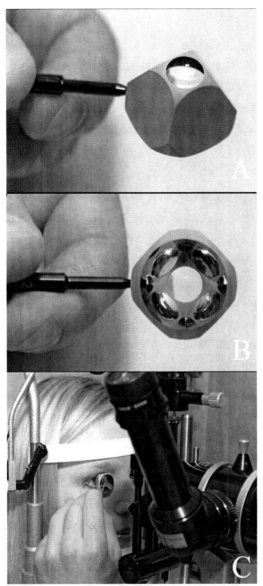

Figure 3-3. Gonioscopy. A and B. The drainage angle is examined using a special lens (gonioscopy lens). C. The gonioscopy lens is gently held against the cornea. Eye doctors look through the gonioscopy lens to see the drainage angle.

3-C. Optic nerve damage

The primary function of the optic nerve is to convey visual signals received by the retina to the brain. As described in Chapter 1, specific sections of the optic nerve are responsible for transmitting particular parts of the visual field to the brain. If part of the optic nerve is damaged by glaucoma, the visual signals from a portion of the visual field are no longer reported to the brain and a blind-spot (called *scotoma*) is formed.

Eye doctors may directly observe the optic nerve damage by looking through the pupil with an ophthalmoscope. A healthy optic nerve is pink, and the ratio of the diameter of the optic cup to that of the optic disc in a healthy eye is generally less than 0.5 (see Chapter 1-B for more discussion). When the optic nerve is damaged many of the individual fibers that make up the nerve are lost and the optic nerve becomes excavated or "cupped." As glaucoma progresses and more optic nerve tissue is lost, the optic cup grows larger (Figure 3-4).

The superior and inferior aspects of the optic nerve are preferentially damaged by glaucoma. These parts of the nerve are responsible for peripheral vision. Consequently, as the optic cup enlarges, it typically becomes vertically elongated. In advanced stages of glaucoma, the portion of the nerve that carries central vision may also become involved.

Bleeding or hemorrhage of the optic nerve is another sign of damage from glaucoma. There is a characteristic appearance to optic nerve hemorrhage that is due to the anatomy of the eye. When optic nerve bleeding occurs in glaucoma, the blood typically collects along the individual nerve fibers that radiate outwards from the nerve (Figure 3-5.) An optic nerve hemorrhage is a sign that glaucoma may not be under good control, and additional therapy may be necessary to bring the glaucoma under control.

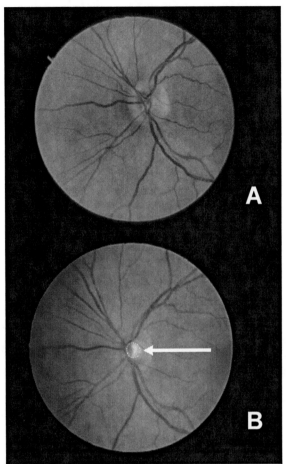

Figure 3-4. Progressive cupping of the optic disc. Early progression of cupping can be seen by comparing sequential photographs of the optic nerve. The optic cup that was initially not visible (A) has enlarged over time (B). The arrow indicates the enlarged cup.

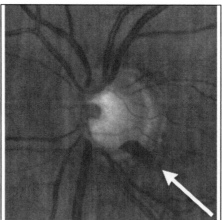

Figure 3-5. Optic nerve hemorrhage. There is a flame-shaped hemorrhage of the optic nerve located at the arrow at 5 o'clock.

The cause of the optic nerve damage in glaucoma is not well understood. In most patients that have elevated intraocular pressure, the progression of glaucoma is halted when the pressure is lowered to a more normal level with medicines or surgery. High intraocular pressure may directly damage the optic nerve and cause vision loss in this subset of patients. In other patients, the optic nerve is injured at pressures that are not elevated (or in the normal range). The optic nerves of these patients (so-called "normal tension glaucoma") appear to be sensitive to damage at intraocular pressures that most people tolerate without any harmful effects. Studies have shown that lowering the intraocular pressure to low normal or even sub-normal levels can halt the progression of normal tension glaucoma. Additional mechanisms such as poor blood circulation to the optic nerve may be responsible for optic nerve damage in normal tension glaucoma.

Chapter 4

4-A. Introduction

The diagnosis of glaucoma has different implications for patients depending on the type of glaucoma diagnosed. Those with suspicious findings for glaucoma are called *glaucoma suspects*. These patients need to be watched carefully for the development of glaucoma. Crossing the line between being a suspect to actually being diagnosed with the disease depends on the development of optic nerve cupping with corresponding visual field loss. There are two categories of glaucoma when the diagnosis is made: open-angle and angle-closure. Different risk factors (see Chapter 5) and treatments exist for each type.

4-B. The Glaucoma Suspect

Patients are also glaucoma suspect if they have elevated intraocular pressure (often referred to as *ocular hypertension*). Normal intraocular pressure is considered 10 to 21 mmHg. Those with ocular hypertension have intraocular pressures greater than 21 mmHg. Accurate intraocular pressure measurement depends on the thickness of the cornea. Thin corneas may underestimate the intraocular pressure measurement since it is easier to press against the cornea when checking the intraocular pressure. Thus when the cornea is thin, the true intraocular pressure is higher than the measured intraocular pressure. Conversely, when the cornea is thick, the true intraocular pressure is lower than the measured intraocular pressure. Corneal thick-

25

ness measurements are made with a pachymeter (Figure 4-2). It is performed with a topical (eye drop). The intraocular pressure measurement is combined with the corneal thickness measurement to ascertain the true level of intraocular pressure (Figure 4-3).

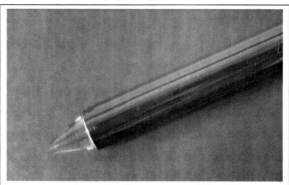

Figure 4-2. A pachymeter tip used to measure corneal thickness.

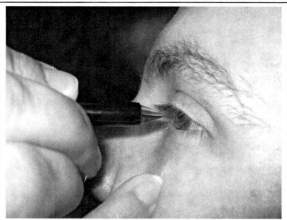

Figure 4-3. A patient undergoes *pachymetry* to determine his corneal thickness.

Despite cupping or high intraocular pressures (IOPs), the visual field test is normal in glaucoma suspects. Progressing to glaucoma requires cupping with corresponding visual field loss. At risk for the progression to glaucoma are those with elevated IOPs, thin corneas (less than 555 microns), African descent, older age, enlarged cups, and a family history of glaucoma.

Optic nerve photographs are helpful in following glaucoma suspects. Comparison of optic nerves to previous photos allows eye doctors to determine if there is progression of optic nerve cupping. Changes in the optic nerve appearance over time indicate glaucomatous damage (see Figure 3-4, page 23). A visual field test which begins to show signs of visual field loss indicates that glaucoma is developing. It is, therefore, important for glaucoma suspects to be carefully monitored with serial eye examinations over time. Since glaucoma often develops without symptoms, the first signs of glaucoma development may be detected on examination by an eye doctor. Screening should be performed every 2 - 4 years after the age of 40 and every 1 - 2 years after the age of 65 (see Chapter 2). Those with more risk factors are examined more frequently than those without risks.

4-C. Open-Angle Glaucoma

One common type of glaucoma is open-angle glaucoma. The difference between open-angle and angle-closure glaucoma is based on examination. The term angle (short for *irido-corneal angle*) refers to the drainage angle of the eye, which is between the cornea and the iris. Those with open-angle glaucoma have a widely open drainage angle on examination. The angle is examined with a special lens called a gonioscopy lens ("gonio" means angle) (Figure 4-4. Also see Figure 3-3, page 21).

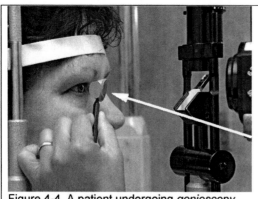

Gonioscopy
Lens

Figure 4-4. A patient undergoing *gonioscopy*

An open-angle with cupping of the optic nerve and glaucomatous visual field loss is consistent with the diagnosis of open-angle glaucoma. There are primary and secondary causes of open-angle glaucoma. If there is no identifiable factor causing the glaucoma (i.e., the cause of the glaucoma is unknown), this is referred to as *primary open-angle glaucoma* (POAG) or chronic open-angle glaucoma (COAG). POAG is the most common form of glaucoma in the United States. Primary open-angle glaucoma can be of two types. It can be associated with either elevated intraocular pressure (IOP) or normal IOP. The former is referred to as POAG with elevated IOP or *high pressure glaucoma*. The latter is referred to as *normal tension glaucoma (NTG)* or low tension glaucoma. NTG has the same characteristics as POAG except the IOP is in the normal range (less than 21 mmHg). One theory regarding the mechanism of injury in NTG is insufficient blood flow leading to optic nerve damage. Although NTG patients have IOPs less than 21 mmHg, it has been shown that lowering the IOP to low-normal or even sub-normal range halts or slows the progression of glaucomatous damage. Aside from the IOP, a few differences have been observed. More optic nerve hemorrhages (bleeding spots) are found in normal tension glaucoma than in patients with high pressure glaucoma. The visual field test may also show more central (as opposed to peripheral) loss in normal tension glaucoma. These differences are not absolute and many of the characteristics between the two forms overlap. If there is a known process leading to decreased fluid drainage through the angle, such as blood, inflammatory cells, or pigment, this is called *secondary open-angle glaucoma.* Glaucomas associated with *pigment dispersion syndrome* and *pseudoexfoliation syndrome* are examples of secondary open-angle glaucoma.

The treatment goal of open-angle glaucoma is to lower intraocular pressure. This is more challenging in normal tension glaucoma (NTG). However, lowering intraocular pressure has been shown to be effective even in NTG as well as high pressure glaucoma. Treatment modalities include topical medications (eye drops), laser to the drainage area or trabecular meshwork (laser trabeculoplasty), and filtering surgery. Medical and surgical treatment will be covered in more depth in Chapters 7 and 8.

4-D. Angle-closure Glaucoma

Angle-closure glaucoma may present very differently from open-angle glaucoma. In contrast to open-angle glaucoma, which is mostly asymptomatic, acute angle-closure glaucoma may present suddenly with pain, nausea, and decreased vision. As the name implies, the drainage angle is closed when examined with a gonioscopy lens.

The mechanism of angle-closure comes from a contact between the lens and iris. Once this contact occurs, aqueous fluid is unable to pass into the anterior chamber through the pupil. This is called *pupillary block* (Figure 4-5).

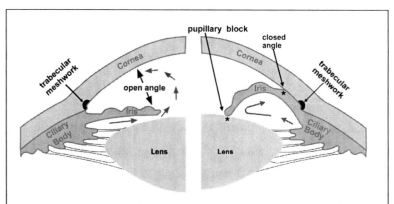

Figure 4-5. An open angle is shown on the left. Aqueous is free to pass between the iris and lens and drain through the trabecular meshwork. *Pupillary block* (angle-closure) is shown on the right. Aqueous is trapped behind the iris which pushes it forward to obstruct the trabecular meshwork.

The aqueous fluid then accumulates behind the iris and pushes the iris forward. The peripheral iris then obstructs the trabecular meshwork or drainage angle. The inability for aqueous to exit the eye causes an elevation in intraocular pressure. This process may occur acutely or chronically. If the pressure rise is sudden, pain occurs. When it happens chronically, it may be less symptomatic. Occasionally the episodes of angle-closure may occur intermittently. In these cases, patients may have episodic symptoms of blurry vision, eye pain, or headache.

The risk factors for angle-closure glaucoma are not the same as in open-angle glaucoma. Those at risk tend to have narrow angles. Patients who are older, female, hyperopic (far-sighted), or from an Asian background tend to be at greater risk for angle-closure glaucoma. Older age tends to be a risk factor because the lens thickens over time leading to a higher likelihood of pupillary block. Hyperopia tends to occur in people with small eyes. These eyes tend to be crowded and more likely to develop pupillary block (see Chapter 5).

For those at risk, pupil dilation may also cause a higher likelihood of angle-closure. Pharmacologic pupil dilation, therefore, is contraindicated in patients with narrow, occludable angles (Figure 4-6). Various over-the-counter and prescription medications are also contraindicated due to the same mechanism. Once definitive treatment (laser peripheral iridotomy) is administered, these medications are no longer contraindicated.

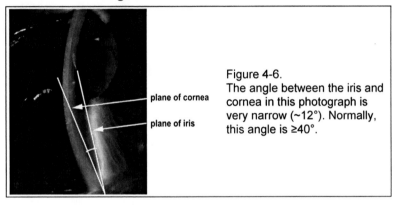

plane of cornea

plane of iris

Figure 4-6.
The angle between the iris and cornea in this photograph is very narrow (~12°). Normally, this angle is ≥40°.

In acute angle-closure glaucoma, a patient may have pain, nausea/vomiting, headache, a red eye, cloudy cornea, a shallow anterior chamber, and elevated intraocular pressure. Glaucoma eye drops are given to decrease the intraocular pressure but a definitive treatment needs to be done to break or relieve the pupillary block. The definitive treatment for acute angle-closure glaucoma is laser peripheral iridotomy (LPI; Figure 4-7). This laser procedure places a hole in the iris to circumvent the pupillary block, thereby allowing the iris to fall back and open up the drainage angle. If a patient cannot sit for a laser procedure, such as in children, a surgical iridectomy may be performed in the operating room under general anesthesia. The same procedure (iridotomy) should eventually be performed in the unaffected fellow eye to prevent a future occurrence in that eye. Once the procedure is performed in both eyes, patients may be dilated or take medications without fear of precipitating acute angle-closure glaucoma.

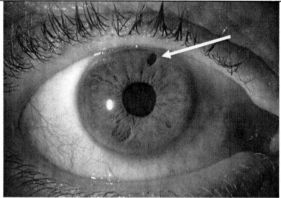

Figure 4-7. Laser peripheral iridotomy (LPI). The laser treatment for acute angle-closure glaucoma creates a small hole in the iris (arrow).

Symptoms of angle-closure may also occur intermittently. In these cases, LPI is beneficial in preventing intermittent attacks of angle-closure. When angle-closure glaucoma is noted in a chronic setting, LPI may or may not be beneficial. In these cases, elevated intraocular pressure may be treated with LPI, topical medications, or filtering surgery.

4-E. Childhood Glaucoma

Although glaucoma occurs mostly in adults, children can get glaucoma as well. Glaucoma that is present at birth or within the first few years of life is called congenital or infantile glaucoma. Congenital glaucoma occurs in 1 of 30,000 live births. It may be inherited or can occur spontaneously without family history. It tends to occur more often in males and does not appear to have racial predilection.

As in adult glaucoma, an elevated intraocular pressure leads to glaucomatous optic nerve damage. The clinical presentation, however, is very different. Unlike in adult glaucoma, infants have eyes which are still growing and elevated intraocular pressure can cause a further increase in the size of their eyes. The enlargement of the eye from congenital glaucoma is called buphthalmos (meaning "ox eye"; Figure 4-8). The high intraocular pressure can also cause their cornea to become cloudy or hazy, which can cause tearing and the sensitivity to light ("photophobia"). One or both eyes may be affected.

Typical findings of congenital glaucoma include buphthalmos (enlarged eye), sensitivity to light, and tearing from the cloudy cornea. The elevated intraocular pressure also causes the posterior layer of the cornea to be torn (Haab's striae), in addition to optic nerve cupping and visual loss. In addition, these children are at high risk for developing "lazy eye" or amblyopia because the impaired vision secondary to cloudy cornea.

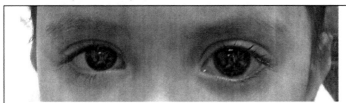

Figure 4-8. The left eye of this congenital glaucoma patient is noticeably larger than the right eye. The patient has buphthalmos of the left eye.

The examination of children with suspected glaucoma includes measurements of the eye length and cornea, intraocular pressure, gonioscopy, as well as dilated examination for evaluation of the optic nerve. This may require that the infant be sedated (or put under general anesthesia) for examination (Figure 4-9). Ultrasound is used for measurements of the eye length. Serial measurements may be made to determine if the eye is stable or becoming too large from high intraocular pressures. Obviously, infants cannot verbalize their visual loss or perform visual field testing. Therefore, their glaucoma is followed with careful eye exams.

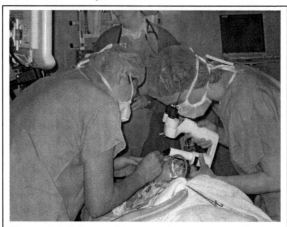

Figure 4-9. Infants with congenital glaucoma often require general anesthesia to perform an adequate examination.

Congenital glaucoma is caused by abnormal development of trabecular meshwork which leads to decreased outflow of aqueous fluid from the eye. Since this developmental abnormality is the cause of the high intraocular pressure, the treatment is aimed towards relieving this abnormality. The treatment is surgical incision of the abnormal trabecular meshwork, which allows better outflow of aqueous fluid from the eye. This is in contrast to adult glaucoma where surgery is often the last line of treatment for glaucoma. In addition, once surgery relieves the elevated intraocular pressure, the optic nerve damage (or cupping) may be reversible; this is in contrast to irreversible nature of optic nerve damage in adult glaucoma (see in Chapter 10).

Despite treatment with surgery to relieve the anatomic abnormality, patients who have had congenital or infantile glaucoma need to be followed chronically for the progression of their disease. They will require periodic eye examination into adulthood.

Chapter 5

Glaucoma Risk Factors

5-A. Risk Factors for Primary Open-angle Glaucoma

Primary open-angle glaucoma (POAG) has several well-known risk factors. They include *elevated intraocular pressure (IOP), older age, black race, and positive family history.*

1) **Elevated Intraocular Pressure (IOP)**: While elevated IOP is not necessary for having glaucoma (for example, normal tension glaucoma), it is clear that elevated IOP increases the chance of developing glaucoma (Table 5-1). For example, if you have an IOP of 30 mmHg, your chance of having glaucoma is 25.4%, and your risk of developing glaucoma is 39 times higher than those with IOP <15mmHg.

Table 5-1. Increasing risk of developing POAG according to increasing intraocular pressure (IOP).

IOP (mmHg)	Prevalence in population (%)	Relative Risk (fold)
<15	0.7	1.0
16-18	1.3	2.0
19-21	1.8	2.8
22-24	8.3	12.8
25-29	8.3	12.8
30-34	25.4	39.0
≥ 35	26.1	40.1

We now know that measurement of intraocular pressure is at least partly dependent on the *corneal thickness*. In thicker corneas, the true intraocular pressure is lower than the measured intraocular pressure; in thinner corneas, the true intraocular pressure is higher than the measured intraocular pressure. Therefore, the measurement of corneal thickness (*pachymetry*) is an important part of measuring intraocular pressure.

2) **Older age**: Like many other diseases, glaucoma occurs more frequently in an older population (Table 5-2). For example, the prevalence of primary open-angle glaucoma (POAG) increases from 0.6% in a 40-year old to 7.3% in an 80 year-old white person. This is > 12 fold increase in risk in the 40-year span.

Table 5-2. Increasing risk of developing POAG according to increasing age and race.				
Age (years)	White	Black	Hispanic	Asian
40-49	0.6	1.2	0.5	0.3
50-59	1.5	4.1	1.6	1.6
60-69	2.7	5.5	1.7	1.8
70-79	5.1	9.2	5.7	2.9
80+	7.3	11.3	12.6	N/A
Overall	N/A	4.7	2.0	1.2

3) **Black race**: The prevalence is generally higher in blacks than in whites (Table 5-2). Hispanics had similar prevalence as whites, except for the oldest age group (80+ years) whose prevalence (12.6%) was higher than in whites and was comparable to that of blacks. Asians had similar prevalence as whites. Blacks are not only more likely to develop glaucoma, they are also more likely to lose sight and become blind once glaucoma develops.

4) **Positive family history of glaucoma**: Like many other diseases, there is hereditary component to glaucoma. If you have a first-degree relative (parent, sibling, or child) with glaucoma, your risk of developing glaucoma is 2-4 times higher than those with-

out family history. This strongly suggests genetic component to the disease. Several genes (and their location in the chromosome or DNA) have been implicated in primary open-angle glaucoma (POAG). The most well-studied is the myocilin gene on chromosome 1, which accounts for 3-5% of POAG patients. Other genes, yet to be discovered, are suspected to play a role in the remaining POAG population (see Chapter 11).

5) Additional minor risk factors for POAG include: *myopia* (nearsightedness), diabetes, and elevated blood pressure. While elevated blood pressure is associated with the increase in the risk of POAG in a population study, there is no direct relationship between the two in individual patients. In other words, the intraocular pressure and blood pressure are not directly correlated (linked) in a given patient. Migraine headaches and *Raynaud's disease* (poor circulation in hands and feet) have been associated with normal tension glaucoma.

5-B. Risk Factors for Primary Angle-Closure Glaucoma

The *primary angle-closure glaucoma* (*PACG*) has several risk factors of its own. They include: older age, Asian race, female gender, hyperopia (far-sightedness), and positive family history.

1) **Older age**: Like primary open-angle glaucoma, the older age increases the risk of primary angle-closure glaucoma. One reason for this may be that as you get older, a *cataract* (cloudy lens) develops which results in thickening and narrowing of the anterior chamber drainage angle (see Chapter 3 for the eye anatomy). The narrow drainage angle predisposes the patient for PACG.

2) **Asian race**: The Asian populations (especially of Far Eastern extraction) are at a higher risk for developing primary angle-closure glaucoma (PACG) than the other races (see Chapter 2, Table 2-3). PACG exists in 0.3 ~ 2.7% of the adult Asian populations, while it exists in only 0.1 ~ 0.6% in other races (white, black and Hispanic adult population). The exact reason for this is unclear. However, smaller anterior chamber depth has been found to be associated with PACG. It is possible that the Asian population as a group has smaller anterior chamber depth than other populations, thus increasing the risk for PACG.

3) **Female gender**: In PACG, females are more common than males. It is generally believed that females (compared to males) have smaller eyes and, therefore, smaller anterior chambers, and narrower drainage angles. These are in turn anatomical risk factors for the development of PACG.

4) **Hyperopia (far-sightedness)**: Like female gender, far-sighted people tend to have smaller eyes compared to near-sighted people. Smaller eyes tend to have smaller anterior chamber depth and narrower drainage angles, increasing the risk of PACG.

5) **Positive family history of primary angle-closure glaucoma (PACG)**: It has been reported that up to 20% of *relatives* of PACG patients have anatomically narrow drainage angles. It is generally believed that the eye size (like height) is inherited. If the small eye size (and, therefore, narrow drainage angle) is inherited, this would explain the inheritability of PACG.

It is important to identify those who are at risk for development of primary angle-closure glaucoma, because the rate of blindness from angle-closure glaucoma is higher than in primary open-angle glaucoma. There are ongoing studies in Asia looking at best ways to screen for primary angle-closure glaucoma in a large population. Until we know better ways to detect primary angle-closure glaucoma early, our recommendation is to seek periodic ophthalmic evaluation by an eye doctor (Table 5-3).

Table 5-3. Recommended frequency of eye examinations by American Academy of Ophthalmology		
Age group	No glaucoma risk factors	Glaucoma risk factors
20-29	At least once during interval	Every 3-5 years
30-39	At least twice during interval	Every 2-4 years
40-64	Every 2-4 years	Every 2-4 years
65+	Every 1-2 years	Every 1-2 years

In those patients who are susceptible for primary angle-closure glaucoma (or have narrow drainage angles), taking certain medications (both prescription and over-the-counter) can precipitate an acute angle-closure glaucoma attack. These medications contain ingredients that tend to dilate the pupil (as a side effect). In susceptible patients with a narrow drainage angle (called an *occludable angle*), the pupil dilation can precipitate an acute angle-closure attack, often raising the intraocular pressure to very high levels (40-50 mmHg are not uncommon). It is important to ask the pharmacist and read the drug label thoroughly before taking these medications. It is important to note that these drugs have no adverse effect in open-angle glaucoma patients. If you are not sure, ask your eye doctor whether you are at risk for development of angle-closure glaucoma before taking the medication. Finally, several classes of drugs have been reported to cause acute angle-closure, even in non-susceptible patients. For example, topiramate (Topamax®) used in seizure and migraine disorders has been reported to cause acute angle-closure glaucoma in patients who are typically not at risk. Other medications associated with angle-closure glaucoma include tricyclic antidepressants, serotonin uptake inhibitors, and diuretics. It is important to monitor for angle-closure glaucoma if you are taking one of these medications.

5-C. Risk factors for childhood glaucoma

Childhood glaucoma usually refers to those that occur very early in life (in the first 3 years of life). It is also commonly referred to as infantile or congenital glaucoma (see Figure 4-8, page 33). When glaucoma occurs between the ages of 3 - 39 years, it is usually referred to as "juvenile" glaucoma.

Infantile glaucoma is a rare disease; it occurs in approximately 1 in 30,000 live births. Infantile glaucoma can occur in isolation, or along with other ocular or systemic abnormalities (for more detail, see Chapter 10). When it occurs in isolation, it is called *primary infantile (or congenital) glaucoma*. Primary infantile glaucoma occurs more commonly in boys than in girls (at the ratio of 3:2); however in Japan the gender ratio may be reversed (2:3 for boys:girls). While most of them occur without family history, approximately 10% have positive family history. If the first child has the disease, the risk of disease for the second child is about 3%. If the first 2 children have the disease, the risk for the third child is up to 25%. Thus, all siblings of an affected child should be examined closely by a pediatric ophthalmologist. Recently, mutations in the *CYP1B1 gene* on chromosome 2 has been found to be associated with congenital glaucoma. In the future, we may discover additional genes responsible for congenital glaucoma.

Juvenile glaucoma presents between the ages of 4 and 39, and usually associated with very high intraocular pressure. They typically have very strong positive family history of glaucoma with several older members of the family having been affected by the disease. Mutations in the gene, *Myocilin* (sometimes called *TIGR*) on chromosome 1, have been found to be associated with patients with juvenile glaucoma. If you have a strong positive family history of infantile or juvenile glaucoma, it would be reasonable to be screened for glaucoma by an eye doctor at a younger age.

Chapter 6

The eye examination and diagnosis

6-A. What to expect

An eye examination to assess for glaucoma is not very different from the standard "check-up" visit conducted by an eye doctor. In fact, many elements of a glaucoma evaluation are routinely conducted at routine visits to an eye doctor. These glaucoma "vital signs" are listed in Table 6-1 and are discussed in detail below. The elements of this examination should not be painful and are well tolerated by most patients.

Table 6-1. Glaucoma "vital signs." The most important elements of a glaucoma examination are shown in this table.

Element of the exam	Purpose
Visual acuity test (reading the eye chart)	Assess central vision
Intraocular pressure (IOP) measurement	Test for pressure within the eye
Gonioscopy	Assess drainage angle (open or closed)
Visual field test	Assess peripheral vision
Optic nerve exam (for cupping)	Assess optic nerve for damage
Imaging Study (color photos, computerized optic nerve analyzers)	Assess health of optic nerve

Some parts of a glaucoma examination are done at every visit, while other parts are evaluated less frequently. Visual acuity, intraocular pressure, and the optic nerve appearance are assessed at every visit, while the drainage angle and peripheral vision are evaluated at regular intervals (typically once a year or so).

Color photographs are taken of the optic nerve using a camera that is focused through the pupil towards the back of the eye. These pictures document the appearance of the optic nerve at a particular time point. The photos are used by the eye doctor to help recognize progressive damage to the nerve (increased cupping) by allowing a comparison of the current optic nerve appearance to a prior photograph.

Specialized imaging devices such as an Optical Coherence Tomograph (OCT, Carl Zeiss Meditec, Dublin, CA), Heidelberg Retinal Tomograph (HRT, Heidelberg Engineering, Inc. Vista, CA), or a scanning laser polarimeter (GDx, Carl Zeiss Meditec, Dublin, CA) may also be used to help assess the health of the optic nerve. These instruments take images of the optic nerve and retina similar to a photographic camera. The images captured by these devices are used to quantify the amount of cupping and thickness of the fibers that make up the optic nerve.

6-B. Intraocular pressure and corneal pachymetry

The normal intraocular pressure (IOP) is between 10 to 21 mmHg. Any intraocular pressure lower than 5 mmHg is considered abnormally low and is referred to as *hypotony*. An intraocular pressure greater than 21 mmHg is considered abnormally high and is often referred to as *ocular hypertension*. High intraocular pressure does not necessarily mean that you have glaucoma. It simply increases the risk for the development of glaucoma. The higher the intraocular pressure, the greater the risk of developing glaucoma (see Chapter 5).

Intraocular pressure is not constant and can vary throughout the day. A diurnal variation is intraocular pressure fluctuation during the day, while a nocturnal variation is fluctuation of intraocular pressure during the night. Sometimes when the eye doctor is suspicious that there is a great fluctuation of intraocular pressure during the day, he may recommend measurement of diurnal intraocular pressures. At the University of Iowa this is performed at 3-hour intervals starting at 7:00AM until 10:00PM as an outpatient. It is not uncommon to see intraocular pressures slightly higher in the morning than in the afternoon or evening. However, this is not necessarily true for all patients. While there is small diurnal fluctuation of intraocular pressure even in normal subjects, the glaucoma patient tends to have higher intraocular pressure and greater fluctuation of intraocular pressure throughout the day compared to normals.

There are a number of ways to measure the intraocular pressure (IOP) (the measurement of IOP is referred to as *tonometry*). A common measurement technique is Goldmann applanation tonometry. With an anesthetic eye drop, this device measures the IOP by putting a biprism plastic tip against the cornea and *applanating* (or flattening) the cornea. The intraocular pressure is read by dialing in an appropriate amount of force to flatten the surface of the cornea. The Gold-

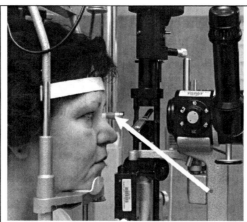

Goldmann Applanation Tip

Figure 6-1. Checking intraocular pressure (IOP) using a Goldmann applanation tip at the slit lamp

mann applanation technique is based on the principle that the force required to flatten a certain defined area of the cornea (which has a curved surface) is proportional to the IOP. (Figure 6-1)

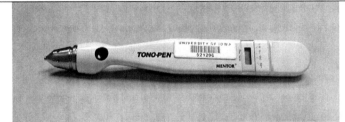

Figure 6-2. Tonopen XL. A hand-held digital device to measure the intraocular pressure. It is useful in patients who are not able to get into the slit lamp for Goldmann applanation tonometry or those with corneal disease.

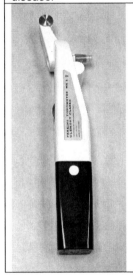

Figure 6-3. Perkins tonometer. It is a hand-held device used to measure the intraocular pressure. It is often used in infants or elderly in a wheelchair. It works on a similar principle as the Goldmann applanation tonometer.

Besides the Goldmann applanation tonometry, there are other devices that can measure the intraocular pressure. Other commonly used tonometers are Tonopen™ (Mentor, Norwell, MA. Figure 6-2) and Perkins (Clement Clarke Inc., Columbus, OH. Figure 6-3) applanation tonometers; both of them are hand-held and portable. These devices come in handy when the patient is unable to easily place the chin at the slit lamp device, as in children or elderly in a wheelchair. Another commonly used device is a non-contact applanation tonometer (commonly referred to as "air puff" tonometer). It is based on a similar principle as the Goldmann applanation tonometry, except that it uses an air puff to flatten the cornea, rather than a direct contact with the tonometer tip. There are do-it-yourself devices such as Proview™ Eye Pressure Monitor (Bausch & Lomb, Rochester, NY) which is available for self-measurement of intraocular pressure at home by the patient. However, the reliability of the home tonometer is considered to be less than the ones commonly used in the doctor's office. Because the home tonometer can sometimes give erroneous readings, eye doctors do not commonly utilize it.

Intraocular pressure reading is performed using a topical anesthesia; it typically takes a few seconds to measure the intraocular pressure in each eye in a cooperative patient. It is painless procedure when performed properly. A complete intraocular pressure assessment requires both the applanation tonometry as well as the corneal thickness measurement.

As discussed in Chapter 4, accurate intraocular pressure measurement depends on the thickness of the cornea. Corneal thickness is measured using a *pachymeter* (Figure 6-4) and the normal corneal thickness is in the range of 0.53 – 0.55 mm. After an anesthetic eye drop is applied, corneal thickness is measured by gently touching the smooth tip of the pachymeter probe to the surface of the cornea (Figure 6-5). With thin corneas, the true intraocular pressure is higher than what is measured using an applanation tonometer. Conversely, in the thicker cornea, the true intraocular pressure is lower than what is measured by applanation tonometry. If you have corneal thickness less than 0.50 or greater than 0.60 mm, the applanation tonometry will significantly underestimate or overestimate the intraocular pressure readings respectively.

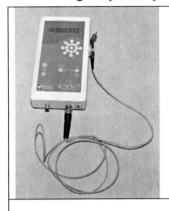

Figure 6-4. Pachymeter. A pachymeter (Pocket Pachymeter, Quantel Medical, Bozeman, MT) is an ultrasound device that measures cornea thickness by determining the time it takes for a sound wave to reflect off the inner surface of the cornea.

Figure 6-5. Pachymetry. Corneal thickness is measured by administering an anesthetic drop to the eye and then gently placing the pachymeter probe against the outer surface of the cornea.

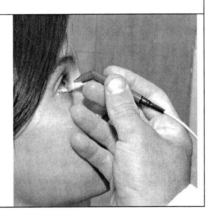

6-C. The drainage angle

Examination of the drainage angle is referred to as *gonioscopy*. The drainage angle is examined to determine if it is *open* or *closed*. To visualize the angle, an anesthetic eye drop is applied to the eye and a special contact lens (gonioscopy lens, Figure 6-6) is placed against the cornea (Figure 6-7). This lens allows an examiner to see into the drainage angle using a slit lamp biomicroscope.

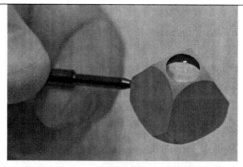

Figure 6-6. A Posner gonioscopy contact lens.

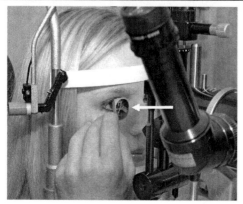

Figure 6-7. Gonioscopy. An examiner gently places the gonioscopy lens (arrow) against the cornea and examines the eye with a slit lamp biomicroscope.

The goal of gonioscopy is to visualize the structures of the drainage angle including the trabecular meshwork (see Chapter 3). Fluid exits the eye through the drainage angle by passing through the trabecular meshwork. If the trabecular meshwork can be seen, the drainage angle is said to be "open". If the drainage angle is obstructed and the trabecular meshwork cannot be visualized, the angle is said to be "closed".

6-D. Optic nerve examination

One of the hallmarks of glaucoma is the optic nerve damage, which is characterized by cupping of the optic nerve. Even a normal

48

optic nerve has a small amount of cupping. However, glaucoma patients tend to have larger cupping than normal subjects. As discussed in Chapter 1, the cup-to-disc ratio of normal subjects is typically around 0.2 to 0.3 (Figure 6-8). The *cup-to-disc ratio* is often measured both in the vertical and horizontal position to estimate the amount of cupping and amount of optic nerve damage (Figure 6-9). The cup size is simply the area of the optic nerve that is not occupied by the optic nerve fibers (an empty space). However, with glaucoma, there is progressive loss of optic nerve fibers, and consequent increase in the cup size of the optic nerve. If the cup-to-disc ratio is 0.3 or less, then this refers to a relatively healthy looking optic nerve. On the other hand, if there is a cup-to-disc ratio close to 1.0, this refers to almost complete cupping and a severely damaged optic nerve from glaucoma (Figure 6-10). While there is no one cup-to-disc ratio that separates normal from glaucoma, the cup-to-disc ratio greater than 0.6 or 0.7 is suspicious of glaucoma and often requires further testing to rule out glaucoma. As glaucoma progresses, the cup-to-disc ratio enlarges (as more optic nerve fiber dies off), and the patient may start to develop peripheral vision loss. A small fraction of glaucoma patients, if detected late or inadequately treated, may become blind in one or both eyes with a complete loss of optic nerve fibers.

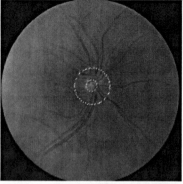

Figure 6-8. Normal optic nerve with a small central cup (0.3 cup-to-disc ratio).

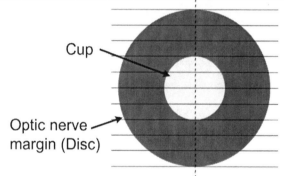

Cup

Optic nerve margin (Disc)

Figure 6-9. The optic nerve is divided into tenths and the cup is compared to the entire optic nerve (optic disc) to obtain the cup-to-disc ratio. The vertical cup-to-disc ratio here is 0.4.

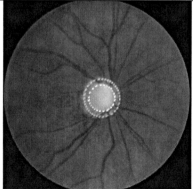

Figure 6-10. Glaucomatous optic nerve with >0.8 cup-to-disc ratio.

In glaucoma the position of the blood vessels within the optic nerve can shift with progressive cupping that can be an important feature of glaucoma progression. Other important optic nerve findings include hemorrhages or bleeding around the optic nerve (Figure 6-11). The optic nerve bleeding is especially common in normal tension glaucoma. It often indicates an ongoing damage to the optic nerve and inadequate control of glaucoma.

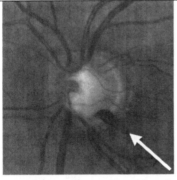

Figure 6-11. Optic nerve hemorrhage. There is a flame-shaped hemorrhage of the optic nerve located at the arrow at 5 o'clock.

Optic nerve can be viewed using a slit lamp with an appropriate lens by an eye doctor. However, in order to objectively document the status of the optic nerve one has to take stereo photographs of the optic nerve, which can be used as a baseline for comparison in the future. Therefore, it is important to take optic nerve photographs at initial exam and periodically afterwards. The stereo photographs of the optic nerve are taken with a "fundus camera" (a camera designed to take pictures of the retina and optic nerve of an eye) in a doctor's office. There are different models of fundus camera, and most fundus cameras can now be modified to take digital pictures (Figure 6-12).

Beginning in the early 1990's, a number of computerized optic nerve imaging devices has been introduced to aid the eye doctor in documenting the optic nerve damage. Currently, these devices in-

51

clude HRT (Heidelberg Retina Tomograph, by Heidelberg Engineering, Inc. Vista, CA, Figure 6-13), Stratus OCT (Optical Coherence Tomography by Carl Zeiss Meditec, Dublin, CA, Figure 6-14), and GDx (or scanning laser polarimeter by Carl Zeiss Meditec, Dublin, CA). These sophisticated instruments provide an accurate map of the optic nerve and quantitative analysis of the optic nerve cupping. In addition, devices such as Stratus OCT and GDx provide the thickness of the nerve fiber layer around the optic nerve, which is related to the amount of cupping. In general, the greater amount of cupping (or the larger the cup-to-disc ratio), the thinner the nerve fiber layer. This is because as you lose more optic nerve fibers, the optic nerve cup gets larger and the nerve fiber layer becomes thinner. Your eye doctor may utilize one or more of these computerized optic analyzers (as well as optic nerve photographs) to evaluate the amount of optic nerve damage in glaucoma to diagnose and follow progression of glaucoma over time. Therefore, it is useful to obtain optic nerve photographs and/or computerized optic nerve imaging on a periodic, ongoing basis. Undoubtedly, there will be improved or new optic nerve imaging devices in the future that may further enhance our ability to diagnose and follow patients with glaucoma.

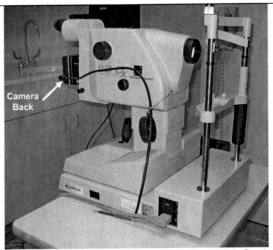

Figure 6-12. A Stereo Disc Fundus Camera (3-Dx, Nidek Co. Ltd, Fremont, CA). A fundus camera such as this is used to take stereo optic nerve photographs of glaucoma patients. It has a digital camera-back which is connected to a computer and hard disc storage device (computer not shown).

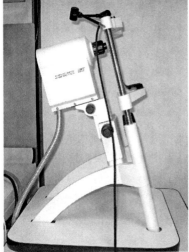

Figure 6-13. Heidelberg Retina Tomograph (HRT). It uses a scanning laser to map out the topography (surface contour) of the optic nerve. The images are then analyzed using a computer to assess the amount of cupping and glaucoma optic nerve damage.

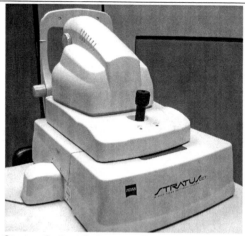

Figure 6-14. Stratus Optical Coherence Tomography (OCT). It uses a coherent laser source to scan a cross-sectional picture of the retina and optic nerve. A computer analysis of the cross-sectional picture allows it to measure the thickness of the nerve fiber layer, which correlates with the amount of cupping and glaucoma optic nerve damage.

6-E. Peripheral vision (visual field testing)

Visual fields measure both central and peripheral vision. Central vision (or "visual acuity") is used for fine-detail tasks such as reading, recognizing faces, and watching television. Peripheral vision is more important for navigating through obstacles in the environment. Early vision loss from glaucoma generally affects peripheral vision. The early peripheral vision loss is not commonly noticed by patients because central vision is usually spared. Therefore, it is important to assess the peripheral vision to detect glaucoma early.

The systematic measurement of visual fields is referred to as *perimetry*. Patients keep one eye fixed on a target directly forward, while the other eye is covered. Next a test object is presented to the test eye at various positions. Patients signal when they see these objects, allowing their visual field to be mapped. Areas in which visual stimuli are not perceived are plotted to indicate the location of visual field defects (blind spot or *scotoma*).

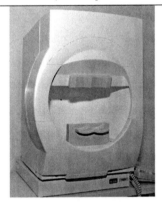

Figure 6-15. Humphrey field analyzer. The Humphrey field analyzer is a commonly used automated perimeter. A computer projects test lights of varying brightness at different positions on the target screen. The visual field is determined by the patient's ability to detect the presence of the test lights.

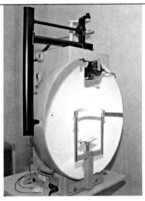

Figure 6-16. Goldmann perimeter. An examiner presents the patient with moving test lights of varying size and brightness to map the visual field .

In glaucoma patients, visual fields are assessed using special devices (*perimeters*) that allow a systematic mapping of blind spots. Patients are placed in front of a bowl-shaped screen and are instructed to indicate when they see test lights that are projected onto various positions on the bowl screen. Some perimeters are computerized and project lights at fixed positions on the screen (Humphrey Field Analyzer, Carl Zeiss Meditec, Dublin, CA, Figure 6-15), while other perimeters are manual and project moving lights on the screen

(Goldmann perimeter, Haag Streit AG, Mason, Ohio Figure 6-16). Patients indicate that they see a target by pressing a button. The output from a Humphrey Field Analyzer is a computer generated plot of the central 24 degrees (Figure 6-17), while the output of the Goldmann perimeter is a manual plotted diagram (Figure 6-18).

Visual field testing requires a high degree of concentration throughout the test. For accurate field measurements, it is important for patients to keep their eye pointed straight ahead at a fixation target while the test lights are presented at various positions on the screen. Visual field testing may take from 5 to 20 minutes per eye depending on type of perimeter and the degree of visual field loss.

Although perimetry provides reliable measurements of visual fields, some variations in the visual fields can occur that are not associated with glaucoma. Consequently, it is often necessary to repeat examinations to confirm the presence of a visual field defect or its progression.

Figure 6-17. Humphrey Field Analyzer visual field reports. These plots represent visual field graphically. The center of the field is at the intersection of the axes. Shading represents areas of vision loss that is proportional to the darkness of the shading.

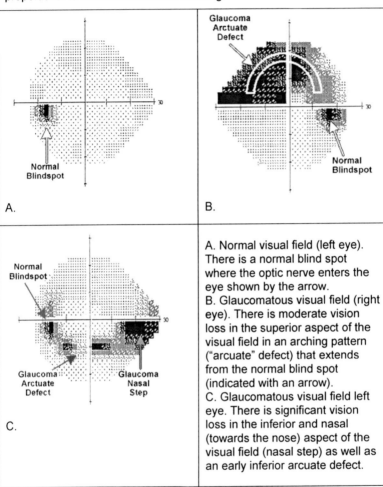

A.

B.

C.

A. Normal visual field (left eye). There is a normal blind spot where the optic nerve enters the eye shown by the arrow.
B. Glaucomatous visual field (right eye). There is moderate vision loss in the superior aspect of the visual field in an arching pattern ("arcuate" defect) that extends from the normal blind spot (indicated with an arrow).
C. Glaucomatous visual field left eye. There is significant vision loss in the inferior and nasal (towards the nose) aspect of the visual field (nasal step) as well as an early inferior arcuate defect.

57

Figure 6-18. Goldmann perimeter visual field reports. The center of the visual field is represented by the intersection of the lines on the grid. Patients are presented with targets of increasing size and brightness. The areas in which these targets can be seen are encircled with colored markings to depict the visual field. Focal areas in which the targets cannot be seen are indicated with color shading using the same color scheme.

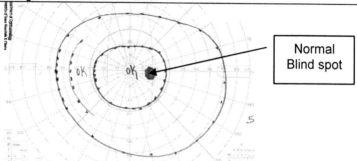

Normal Blind spot

A. Normal visual field. A normal Goldmann visual field (right eye) consists of concentric circular markings. The circular markings (called "isopters") indicate that larger, brighter targets can be seen farther into the periphery than the smaller, dimmer targets. The normal blind spot is shown with an arrow.

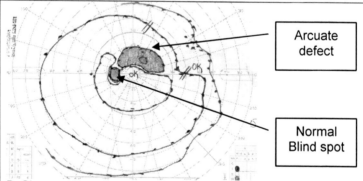

Arcuate defect

Normal Blind spot

B. Glaucomatous visual field (left eye). There is an arc-shaped loss of superior visual field (arcuate defect) that extends from the normal blind spot (indicated with an arrow). This is a typical pattern of vision loss in glaucoma that spares central vision (marked with "OK").

Chapter 7

Medical Treatment of Glaucoma

The purpose of glaucoma treatment is to halt or slow down the progression of nerve damage. Because the optic nerve damage from glaucoma is irreversible, using glaucoma medications will not improve vision or restore visual loss. Glaucoma is treated by lowering the intraocular pressure (IOP). The goal intraocular pressure (or "*target IOP*") for treatment depends on the individual eye and the status of optic nerve damage. Some patients may sustain nerve damage with IOP in the 20s (mm Hg) while others have worsening with the IOP in the teens. Treatment should be tailored toward stabilization of an individual's glaucoma status. Most medical treatments for glaucoma involve eye drops (topical medications). Occasionally oral medications are also used to lower IOP.

7-A. Aqueous Production and Outflow

Changes in intraocular pressure are made by regulating aqueous fluid ("*aqueous humor*") production or drainage. Aqueous fluid is made in the ciliary body and travels between the iris and lens, and through the pupil. It then enters the anterior chamber and drains in the drainage angle (trabecular meshwork, see Figure 7-1). Medications either decrease the production of aqueous fluid (*aqueous suppressants*) or facilitate its outflow from the eye (*outflow drugs*) to lower the intraocular pressure. There are two main outflow passages from the eye: the conventional outflow and non-conventional outflow. The conventional outflow provides a majority of the aqueous drainage through the trabecular meshwork. The non-conventional outflow, or *uveoscleral outflow*, provides the remaining aqueous outflow through the ciliary body face and iris. Outflow drugs may affect one or the other outflow pathways to lower intraocular pressure.

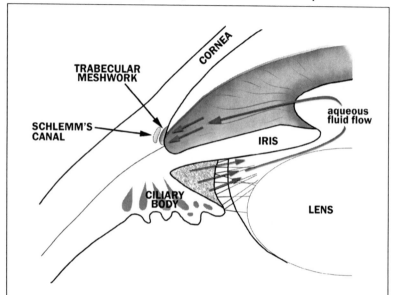

Figure 7-1. Aqueous Fluid Flow in the Eye. The aqueous fluid that fills the eye is produced by the ciliary body and flows between the iris and lens, through the pupil and to the drainage angle at the junction of the iris and the cornea. Aqueous fluid exits the eye through a tissue called the trabecular meshwork in the drainage angle.

7-B. Topical Glaucoma Medications

Currently, there are 5 main classes of topical medications for the treatment of glaucoma. They either lower aqueous production (*aqueous suppressants*) or increase its outflow (*outflow drugs*) (Table 7-1). Some medications may have effect on both. Each class of eye drops can be identified by its cap color (Table 7-2).

Table 7-1. Mechanisms of Glaucoma Medication	
Decrease aqueous fluid production	Increase aqueous fluid outflow
Beta-blockers	Cholinergics
Alpha-adrenergics	Prostaglandin analogs
Carbonic anhydrase inhibitors	

The choice among the various treatments depends upon a patient's health and ocular history. Although these medications are administered topically on the eye, they can have both ocular and systemic side effects. As with any medication, allergies or intolerances may develop with continued use. Common signs and symptoms of allergy are redness, itching, burning, and swelling. If any of these develop, the treating doctor should be contacted and alternative treatments should be discussed.

Table 7-2. Eye drop cap color according to medication class	
Class of Medication	Eye Drop Cap Color
Prostaglandins	Clear/teal
Beta-blockers	Yellow, blue
Alpha-adrenergics	Purple
Carbonic anhydrase inhibitors	Orange
Cholinergics	Green

7-C. Glaucoma Medication Classes

7-C(1). Prostaglandin Analogs

Prostaglandins are chemicals made within the tissues of the body. Receptors exist for each of the various prostaglandins and have different physiologic effects on the body. When activated by prostaglandin PGF2α, the non-conventional outflow (uveoscleral outflow) is improved with resulting decrease in intraocular pressure.

Latanoprost (Xalatan®, Figure 7-2 A) was the first prostaglandin analog developed for the treatment of glaucoma and has been shown to effectively lower intraocular pressure with once daily dosing at bedtime. It is suggested that unopened bottles of latanoprost be refrigerated; once open, they can be stored at room temperature. Travoprost (Travatan®, Figure 7-2 B) and bimatoprost (Lumigan®, Figure 7-2 C), are similar agents that lower intraocular pressure with once daily dosing as well. Unoprostone (Rescula®) is another prostaglandin analog; it is dosed twice daily.

Figure 7-2. Prostaglandin Analogs

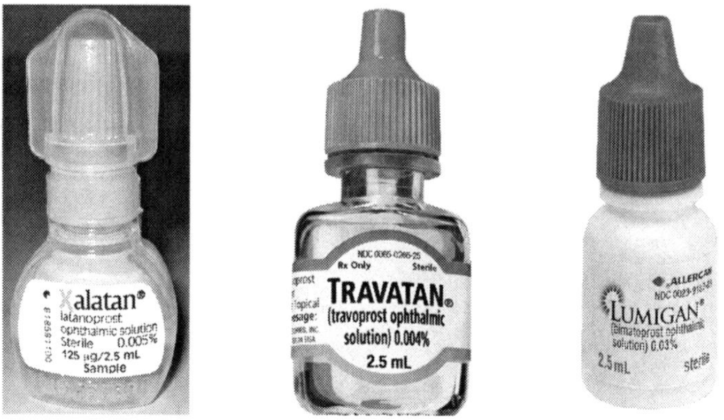

| A. Latanoprost 0.005% (Xalatan®, Pfizer Inc., New York, NY) | B. Travoprost 0.004% (Travatan®, Alcon Inc., Fort Worth, TX) | C. Bimatoprost 0.03% (Lumigan®, Allergan Inc., Irvine, CA) |

Prostaglandins are becoming important first line agents in the treatment of glaucoma. They are well-tolerated and lack significant systemic side effects. They have the added benefit of once daily dosing.

Ocular side effects of prostaglandin analogs include redness, irritation, corneal toxicity (especially in those with a history of herpes simplex keratitis), inflammation, increased pigmentation of periocular skin, iris darkening (especially in hazel/green eye color), and increased length and number of eyelashes. As noted in Table 7-3, the side effects of prostaglandins are primarily ocular. The ocular side effects are not typically severe. The redness and irritation that occur initially tend to improve with time. There is no significant systemic side effect from prostaglandins.

Table 7-3. Ocular side effects of prostaglandins:
Redness
Irritation
Exacerbation of herpes simplex keratitis
Inflammation
Change of periocular skin/iris color
Increased length and number of lashes

7-C(2). Beta-blockers

Beta-adrenergic blockers (beta-blockers) and alpha-adrenergic agonists (see below) work to lower intraocular pressure by affecting the autonomic (or sympathetic) nervous system. The autonomic nervous system exists throughout the body interacting with alpha or beta receptors on cell membranes. Blockers inhibit the action at the receptor while agonists stimulate it. The effects are numerous but in the eye, the main effects are on aqueous production and pupillary constriction/dilation. The two main adrenergic receptors are the alpha and beta receptors. Within each class of receptor, there are subclasses having specific effects. Some medications are selective, meaning that they affect a specific subclass only, while others are nonselective, and they affect the entire class as a whole.

Beta blockers lower intraocular pressure by decreasing the production of aqueous. The most commonly used beta-blocker eye drop is timolol (brand name: Timoptic®, Timoptic XE®, Betimol®, Istalol®). The usual concentrations are 0.25% and 0.5%. It is well tolerated and used either once or twice daily. It comes in both liquid and gel forms. The gel form typically is dosed once daily but has the disadvantage of causing transient blurring of vision. Timolol is easily identified by its cap color of yellow.

Beta-blocker eye drops (brand names in parenthesis) approved for glaucoma treatment include timolol (Timoptic®, Betimol®, Istalol®), levobunolol (Betagan®), carteolol (Ocupress®), metopranolol (OptiPranolol®) and betaxolol (Betoptic®).

Timolol is the most commonly used nonselective beta-blocker and blocks both the $beta_1$ and $beta_2$ receptors. Stimulation of the $beta_1$ receptor increases cardiac contractility, and the $beta_2$ receptor affects bronchodilation. A nonselective blocker inhibits cardiac contractility and bronchodilation. These are, therefore, contraindicated in patients with asthma, emphysema, chronic obstructive pulmonary disease (COPD), bradycardia (low pulse rate), and congestive heart failure. Topical beta blockers have been widely used for glaucoma treatment since early 1980's due to their efficacy. Studies have noted systemic side effects from absorption into the bloodstream from topical application of timolol. Topical beta-blockers may lose their effectiveness over time (tachyphylaxis) in some patients. If this occurs, another medication may be used to control the intraocular pressure. Other nonselective beta-blockers include levobunolol (Betagan®), metipranolol (OptiPranolol®), and carteolol (Ocupress®). Still other beta-blockers are selective for a specific beta receptor. Betaxolol (Betoptic®) is a selective $beta_1$ receptor antagonist. Its mechanism of action is similar to timolol, but since it is a selective $beta_1$ blocker, it is better tolerated in patients with pulmonary disease.

Oral beta-blockers are often used for cardiovascular reasons. Concurrent use of oral beta-blockers may reduce the efficacy of the topical beta blocker. Beta blockers are usually well tolerated. The ocular side effects include redness, burning, decreased corneal sensation, and inflammation. The main systemic side effects include decreased heart rate (bradycardia) and cardiac contractility, irregular heart rhythms (arrhythmias), worsening of congestive heart failure, bronchospasm, difficulty breathing, masking of low blood sugar in diabetics, and depression (Table 7-4). If any of the side effects occur with administration of beta-blocker eye drops, the prescribing doctor should be contacted.

Table 7-4. Side Effects of Beta-Blockers.

Ocular	Systemic
Redness	Bradycardia (low pulse rate)
Burning	Arrhythmias (Irregular pulse)
Decreased corneal sensation	Worsening of congestive heart failure
	Bronchospasm
	Masking of hypoglycemic (low glucose level) symptoms in diabetics
	Depression

7-C(3). Alpha-Adrenergic Agonists

Stimulation of the alpha$_1$-adrenergic receptor produces dilation of the pupil, and the alpha$_2$ receptor decreases aqueous production at the ciliary body. They inhibit the production of aqueous, but they can also facilitate the outflow of aqueous from the eye. Both mechanisms act to lower the intraocular pressure. Alpha$_2$-specific adrenergic agents include brimonidine (Alphagan®, Alphagan-P®) and apraclonidine (Iopidine®). Older, non-specific adrenergic agents include epinephrine and dipivefrin (Propine®). Dipivefrin is a "pro-drug" which is converted in the eye into epinephrine, but the non-specific adrenergic agonists such as dipivefrin are rarely used today.

The specific alpha$_2$-adrenergic agonists, such as brimonidine or apraclonidine, are better tolerated compared to the older nonspecific adrenergic agents. Apraclonidine (Iopidine®) was initially reported to be effective for the treatment of short-term intraocular pressure elevations after ocular laser procedures. Brimonidine is the second generation of alpha$_2$-agonists and has largely replaced apraclonidine. A common side effect of brimonidine is redness and ocular allergy. Alphagan-P® contains a different preservative (Purite®) which helps reduce the preservative-related allergy. Brimonidine is effective in lowering intraocular pressure. Common ocular side effects include allergic symptoms of redness, itching, and irritation. Pupillary dilation and upper lid retraction are also seen. Systemic side effects are uncommon but can include sedation, headache, and fatigue. **Brimonidine should not be used in children under the age of 2** and should be used with caution under the age of 5 due to respiratory and central nervous system depression (Table 7-5). It is contraindicated in patients taking monoamine oxidase inhibitors due to drug interactions.

Table 7-5. Side effects of Alpha$_2$-agonists.

Ocular	Systemic
Redness	Hypotension (low blood pressure)
Itching	**Respiratory depression (especially in infants)**
Irritation	**Central nervous system depression (especially in infants)**
Pupil dilation	Sedation
Lid retraction	Fatigue

7-C(4). Carbonic Anhydrase Inhibitors (CAIs)

The topical carbonic anhydrase inhibitors include dorzolamide (Trusopt®) and brinzolamide (Azopt®). Both are much better tolerated than the systemic CAIs due to reduced side effects. Both are dosed either two or three times daily. In addition, dorzolamide also comes in a combined form with timolol (Cosopt®, Figure 7-3) for better compliance in administration. The CAIs inhibit the enzyme carbonic anhydrase, which in turn, reduces aqueous humor formation. Patients are typically placed on topical glaucoma medications prior to resorting to oral CAIs due to increased systemic side effects associated with oral CAIs. Topical CAIs are effective at lowering the intraocular pressure. They are well-tolerated and have limited systemic side effects. Ocular side effects include irritation, redness, bitter taste after administration, and corneal toxicity. Although much less frequent compared with systemic carbonic anhydrase inhibitors, they may produce a bitter taste and low blood cell counts (Table 7-6).

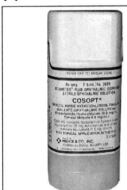

Figure 7-3. Combination beta-blocker and carbonic anhydrase inhibitor: timolol maleate/dorzolamide hydrochloride (Cosopt®, Merck Co., Whitehouse Station, NJ).

Table 7-6. Side Effects of Topical Carbonic Anhydrase Inhibitors.

Ocular	Systemic
Stinging	Allergic symptoms
Irritation	Bitter taste with administration
Redness	Low blood counts
Corneal toxicity	

The carbonic anhydrase inhibitors can be administered systemically (orally). Acetazolamide (Diamox®) and methazolamide (Neptazane®, GlaucTabs®) are the two oral CAIs which may be used for the treatment of glaucoma. Methazolamide is usually better tolerated with fewer side effects than acetazolamide. Reported side effects of oral CAIs include tingling of fingers/toes (*paresthesias*), urinary frequency, electrolyte imbalances, fatigue, anorexia, depression, low potassium levels (*hypokalemia*), poor taste, nausea, diarrhea, kidney stone formation (*nephrolithiasis*), and low blood cell counts. Systemic CAIs are contraindicated in those with an allergy to sulfa, since it is a sulfonamide drug, and in those with a history of renal disease, kidney stones, low potassium (especially in those taking thiazide diuretics), or abnormal blood counts. Oral CAIs may exacerbate these conditions, and should be used with caution (Table 7-7).

Table 7-7. Systemic Side Effects of Systemic Carbonic Anhydrase Inhibitors.
Tingling of fingers/toes (paresthesia)
Urinary frequency
Electrolyte imbalances
Fatigue
Depression
Low potassium levels
Metallic taste
Nausea
Diarrhea
Kidney stone formation
Abnormal blood counts

7-C(5). Cholinergic Agents

The cholinergic agonists act at a receptor called the muscarinic receptor. Once the receptor is activated, the outflow of aqueous through trabecular meshwork is increased. The pupil also constricts (*miosis*). Agents within this class can act directly at the receptor or indirectly by inhibiting the breakdown of the neurotransmitter acetylcholine by the enzyme acetylcholinersterase. The topical medications within this class include pilocarpine, echothiophate iodide, and carbachol. With the number of better tolerated and more easily administered glaucoma drops on the market, these agents are less frequently used today.

Direct-Acting Cholinergic - Pilocarpine

Pilocarpine (Figure 7-4) is a direct-acting cholinergic agonist. It opens the drainage angle and increases the trabecular meshwork aqueous outflow. There are different percentages of pilocarpine, and it has been noted that darker eye colors may require higher dosages of the medication. Dosing is four times daily. Pilocarpine has many ocular side effects (Table 7-8) but systemic side effects are uncommon.

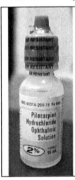

Figure 7-4. Pilocarpine HCl 2% solution. Pilocarpine (a cholinergic agent) constricts the pupil and lowers the intraocular pressure.

Table 7-8. Side effects of pilocarpine.

Ocular	Systemic (uncommon)
Ciliary muscle spasm (eye ache)	Headache
	Perspiration
Pupillary constriction	Increased bronchial secretions
Retinal detachment (rare)	Worsening of Alzheimer's
Corneal toxicity	disease
Inflammation	Stimulation of salivary, lacrimal, gastrointestinal glands

Indirect-Acting Cholinergics – Carbachol, Echothiophate Iodide

Carbachol is both a direct and indirect-acting agent which is used as a topical medication. Echothiophate iodide (Phospholine Iodide®) is an indirect-acting agent which inhibits acetylcholinesterase. The side effects of carbachol are similar to pilocarpine. Both carbachol and echothiophate iodide are rarely used today due to more easily tolerated agents on the market. Occasionally patients will continue on these medications if they were previously started on them with good success and tolerance. A potentially serious complication of echothiophate iodide is pseudocholinesterase depletion. Echothiophate iodide inhibits pseudocholinesterase which breaks down succinylcholine, a paralytic medication sometimes used for general anesthesia. Therefore there can be prolonged respiratory paralysis if used prior to general anesthesia. Therefore, it is important to notify your surgeon and anesthesiologist if you are on these medications before undergoing general anesthesia. Other side effects include nausea, diarrhea, cataracts, iris cysts, and ocular inflammation (Table 7-9).

Table 7-9. Side effects of echothiophate iodide.	
Ocular	Systemic
Ciliary muscle constriction	Headache
Pupillary constriction	Respiratory depression
Retinal detachment	Nausea
Cataract formation	Diarrhea
Iris cysts	Abdominal cramping
Corneal toxicity	Malaise
Inflammation	Prolonged paralysis by succinylcholine during general anesthesia

7-D. Using Glaucoma Medications

Once a decision is made to initiate glaucoma treatment, often a glaucoma medication is tried in one eye only to see if there is an effect. If there is a documented effect in the treated eye, then the medication is added to the fellow eye if necessary. By doing this *one-eye trial*, the untreated eye is used as a control and serves as a basis for comparison to see if the treated eye actually had any effect from the medication. The reason for the one-eye trial is that there is a diurnal fluctuation of intraocular pressure throughout the day. However, the intraocular pressures tend to fluctuate together between fellow eyes. The one-eye medication trial takes advantage of this fact and uses the untreated eye as the control for the treated eye. If there is no effect, another medication is tried. If there is an effect but the intraocular pressure still needs to be lower, another medication may be added.

Practice with instilling eye drops improves the success of administering them correctly (Figure 7-5). The eye can normally hold 7 - 9 μl, and the average drop from an eye dropper is 39 μl. If half of the eye drop fails to stay in the eye, there is still enough retained in the eye to be absorbed. If multiple eye drops are being applied to the same eye, it is best to wait at 10 - 20 minutes between eye drops to enhance drug absorption. Another way to improve absorption (and to decrease the systemic side effect) is to occlude the tear drainage from the eye by punctal occlusion (Figure 7-6). This is performed by pressing on the tear ducts near the inner lower corner of the eyes for several minutes. Eyelid closure for several minutes after eye drop instillation is also helpful in decreasing systemic side effects.

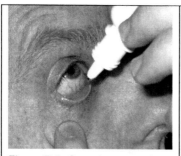 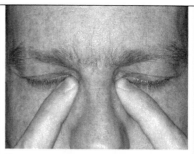

| Figure 7-5. One glaucoma drop is placed on the eye while retracting the lower eyelid. | Figure 7-6. Simple eyelid closure or occlusion of the tear drainage system (punctual occlusion) helps improve ocular absorption while minimizing systemic absorption. |

If maximum glaucoma medications fail to sufficiently lower the intraocular pressure, then laser or surgical treatment can be considered. The surgical treatment options are based on the stage and type of glaucoma.

Chapter 8

Surgical Treatment of Glaucoma

8-A. Glaucoma Laser Treatment

When medications fail to control glaucoma, laser and surgical treatments are often employed. Under appropriate circumstances, surgical treatment can be considered before medical treatment as well.

8-A(1). Laser Trabeculoplasty

Laser trabeculoplasty delivers laser energy to the trabecular meshwork. The goal of treatment is to facilitate the outflow of aqueous humor from the eye in order to lower the intraocular pressure (IOP). The exact mechanism of lowering IOP is not completely understood. It is thought that the laser energy causes cellular changes within the drainage angle, which leads to increased aqueous outflow.

Certain patients have better results with laser trabeculoplasty than others. Patient selection is based on the type of glaucoma and trabecular meshwork pigmentation (coloring). Angle-closure glaucoma is usually not treated with laser trabeculoplasty because the angle cannot be visualized for treatment. In addition, those with narrow angles may develop scarring between the cornea and iris with this type of laser treatment which can further close the drainage angle and exacerbate glaucoma. Therefore, laser trabeculoplasty is usually reserved for the open-angle glaucoma patient. Patients with primary open-angle, pigmentary, or pseudoexfoliation glaucoma tend to do well with laser trabeculoplasty. Some forms of open-angle glaucoma, such

73

as glaucoma from trauma may not respond as well as primary open-angle glaucoma. In addition, laser trabeculoplasty is usually avoided in patients with active inflammation, as in uveitic glaucoma, since it can induce further inflammation.

The trabecular meshwork should be examined by gonioscopy (see Chapter 6-C). More densely pigmented trabecular meshworks respond better to laser since pigment facilitates the uptake of laser energy (e.g., pigmentary and pseudoexfoliation glaucoma). Lightly pigmented trabecular meshworks may require more laser energy, and may be less successful. The optimal candidate is a patient with an open angle with a densely pigmented trabecular meshwork. The eye should be quiet without inflammation. The pre-operative intraocular pressure should not be too high since one of the risks of laser trabeculoplasty is a post-operative intraocular pressure spike due to transient inflammation. Those with end-stage glaucoma may not be able to tolerate the potential post-laser IOP elevation, and instead may require a filtering surgery (see below).

Argon laser trabeculoplasty (ALT) is a common glaucoma laser surgery, which is performed in an office setting. It uses an argon laser which delivers energy in blue-green wavelengths (Figure 8-1). A topical glaucoma eye drop (e.g. brimonidine) is given 15 minutes prior to the procedure to prevent a post-laser IOP elevation. The procedure itself usually takes less than 10 minutes. Patients may experience little or no discomfort during the procedure. Once the eye is anesthetized with a topical eye drop, a contact lens is placed on the surface of the cornea (Figure 8-2). The gonioscopic contact lens allows visualization of the drainage angle. The laser spots are then delivered to the trabecular meshwork. Either 180° (half) or 360° (full) of the angle is treated per treatment session. Each area of the angle is usually treated once to avoid scar formation in the angle.

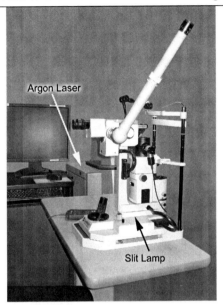

Figure 8-1.
Slit lamp with argon laser used for laser trabeculoplasty.

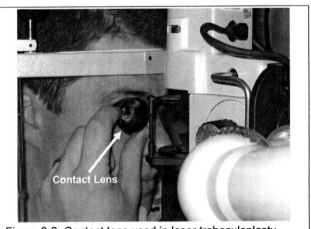

Figure 8-2. Contact lens used in laser trabeculoplasty.

After the laser procedure, another glaucoma eye drop (e.g. bri-monidine) is administered to prevent a post-operative intraocular pressure spike. The intraocular pressure is measured 1 hour after the procedure to ensure that it is stable. Patients are advised to continue the glaucoma medications that they were using prior to the laser treatment. In addition, a short course of topical steroids is given to reduce post-operative inflammation. Patients return for follow-up examination in 4-6 weeks to determine if the ALT treatment decreased the intraocular pressure.

Success rates of the ALT vary. Overall success rate is approximately 50% over 5 years. After this time, many patients require additional intervention to control their intraocular pressure.

Complications of ALT

The most common complication after ALT is the post-laser intraocular pressure spike. Fortunately, the pressure elevation is often transient and rarely causes long-term complication. This occurs from the inflammation that ensues after laser energy is delivered to the trabecular meshwork. It is treated with additional glaucoma medications as needed. Mild anterior segment inflammation (*iritis*) is common after ALT. Post-laser topical steroids are given to control inflammation. Topical steroids are used for 1 to 2 weeks after treatment. Scarring between the iris and the angle (*peripheral anterior synechiae*) may develop after the laser, as well as changes to the peripheral cornea. However, this complication is uncommon in eyes with open angles.

Selective Laser Trabeculoplasty (SLT)

Another similar glaucoma laser procedure is selective laser trabeculoplasty (SLT). This procedure utilizes a neodynium:YAG laser. Unlike ALT, SLT allows the surgeon to repeat the laser surgery over the same area of the angle because the laser targets only the pigmented cells in the trabecular meshwork, while sparing the nonpigmented cells from a thermal damage. Otherwise, the procedure is very similar to ALT. Either 180° or 360° of the angle is treated. It is performed in an office setting with administration of a glaucoma drop (e.g. brimonidine) before and after the procedure, much like the ALT.

Potential complications of SLT are similar to ALT. There is the possibility of post-laser intraocular pressure elevation, which is minimized by the administration of glaucoma drops at the time of the laser treatment. An intraocular pressure check is performed one hour after the procedure. Patients are again advised to continue their previous glaucoma medications and are given a short course of topical steroids.

8-A(2). Laser Peripheral Iridotomy (LPI)

Patients with narrow, occludable angles or who have an attack of acute angle-closure glaucoma are treated with laser peripheral iridotomy (LPI). LPI is done to create a bypass channel for aqueous to flow from behind the iris to the front of the iris, and then, into the drainage angle (see Chapter 4-D). Prior to the advent of laser, a surgery was necessary to create this bypass (*surgical iridectomy*). Currently, a hole is made in the peripheral part of the iris using laser. The procedure is well-tolerated by patients under topical anesthesia. Different lasers are utilized for this procedure including the argon and YAG laser. Sometimes a combination of the two lasers is used to create the LPI. The argon laser typically requires pigment for the uptake of the laser energy and therefore, is better for darker colored (i.e., brown) eyes. The YAG laser disrupts the tissue and can be used in all iris colors.

The LPI typically lasts 10-15 minutes. Prior to the procedure a glaucoma medication (e.g. brimonidine) is given to prevent any post-laser intraocular pressure elevation. In addition, pilocarpine (cholinergic agent – see Chapter 7-C(5)) is given to make the pupil smaller so that the hole can be placed peripherally.

LPI is done under topical anesthesia. A special iridotomy contact lens (Figure 8-3) is placed on the cornea. The laser is then performed through the contact lens. After the procedure, another glaucoma medication (e.g. brimonidine) is given. An intraocular pressure check is performed 1 hour after the laser treatment. Topical steroids are given for several days and then tapered or discontinued. This helps alleviate any inflammation from the laser. The inflammatory cells and pigment released during iridotomy may cause decreased vision after the laser, but this typically subsides within a week.

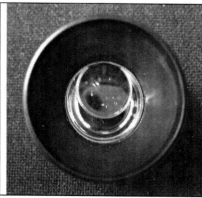

Figure 8-3. Contact Lens for laser iridotomy. This lens allows a magnified view of the iris architecture for laser peripheral iridotomy.

The LPI will relieve intraocular pressure elevation resulting from acute angle-closure glaucoma (see Chapter 9). In cases of narrow, occludable angles with normal intraocular pressure, it will *prevent* acute angle-closure from occurring in the future. Once the iridotomy is made, it remains open and the risk of acute angle-closure glaucoma is eliminated. Even with patent iridotomy hole, patients may still develop intraocular pressure from other mechanisms. These patients are sometimes referred to have *mixed mechanism* glaucoma. The mechanism is mixed because there is a component of both closed- and open-angle contributing to the development of glaucoma.

Complications of LPI

The most frequent complication of LPI is a transient intraocular pressure increase. It is uncommon due to do the use of pre- and post-laser glaucoma medication (e.g. brimonidine). Ocular inflammation, or iritis, may also develop. This is treated with a short course of topical steroids. Ongoing inflammation may sometimes cause closure of the iridotomy site. Corneal or lens damage may occur with the laser treatment due to the proximity of these structures to the peripheral iris. In addition, retinal damage from the laser may rarely occur. Bleeding can occur during the LPI when iris blood vessels are disrupted during the laser procedure. It can be managed by applying gentle pressure with the iridotomy lens, or by simply waiting until blood coagulates on its own. A significant amount of bleeding in the anterior chamber may occasionally cause the intraocular pressure to increase. Rarely, patients may complain of double vision (*diplopia*) or seeing a line in their vision. These visual aberrations may be from the iridotomy hole itself. The symptoms are often transient and become less noticeable over time.

8-A(3). Laser Iridoplasty

After LPI relieves the pupillary block (Chapter 4-D), a narrow angle will usually deepen when observed through a gonioscopy lens. If it does not, a patient may have a condition called *plateau iris* configuration. Plateau iris is caused by a forward rotation of the ciliary body, which causes narrowing of the drainage angle peripherally. Since the condition is not caused by pupillary block, the angle will not deepen after the LPI. To open the peripherally narrow angle, an *iridoplasty* (or *gonioplasty*) may be performed. This procedure uses argon laser to shrink the peripheral iris, which pulls iris away from the trabecular meshwork, opens up the drainage angle, and improves the aqueous outflow.

Iridoplasty is similar to the other laser procedures with regard to intra- and post-operative care. Topical anesthesia is used as well as a glaucoma medication (e.g. brimonidine) to prevent post-laser intraocular pressure (IOP) elevation. A contact lens (Figure 8-4) can be used to visualize the peripheral iris and its contraction with argon laser energy. The laser treatment is usually well-tolerated by patients. Another glaucoma drop is placed post-operatively and the IOP is checked one hour post-operatively to rule out IOP spike. A short course of topical steroids is prescribed. The complications are similar to those of the other ocular laser procedures.

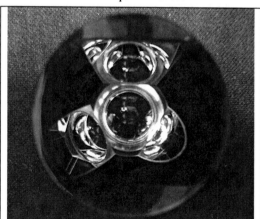

Figure 8-4. Goldmann Contact Lens used for laser iridoplasty. This lens is the same as the one used for laser trabeculoplasty.

8-B. Trabeculectomy: A filtering procedure

It is important to remember that glaucoma surgery lowers intraocular pressure (IOP) to prevent further loss of vision, *not* to improve vision. Lowering the IOP to the target level helps to slow down or halt the progression of optic nerve damage and prevent further loss of vision. Currently, it is not possible to recover lost vision or reverse optic nerve damage from glaucoma; vision loss from glaucoma is, therefore, irreversible. When medications or laser treatment fail to control the intraocular pressure (IOP) in glaucoma, the next step in the management of glaucoma often involves *trabeculectomy*, which is often referred to as a *filtering procedure*.

Preoperative Considerations

Trabeculectomy is a commonly performed glaucoma surgical procedure when medications fail to adequately control the intraocular pressure. It can be performed for most (but not all) types of glaucoma. It is necessary to have intact, non-scarred *conjunctiva*. The conjunctiva is a thin tissue that coats the surface of the *sclera* or eye wall. Trabeculectomy can be difficult to perform in an eye that has had previous ocular surgeries with scarred tissue. In this situation, the surgeon may elect to perform a tube shunt (or *seton*) procedure (see next section).

Anesthesia

The surgery uses a local anesthesia to the eye. Traditionally, a *retrobulbar* (behind the eye) anesthetic injection has been used for local anesthesia. This involves injecting a small amount of anesthetic behind the eye under light intravenous sedation. Retrobulbar anesthesia works well not only in trabeculectomy but in many other types of ocular surgery. However, it can be occasionally associated with serious complications such as *hemorrhage* (bleeding) or even perforation of the eye. In certain cooperative patients, a topical (eye drop) anesthesia can be used to perform trabeculectomy rather than the retrobulbar injection anesthesia. The advantage of the topical anesthesia is quicker visual recovery and decreased risk associated with retrobulbar injection. The surgery is usually done on an outpatient basis.

Surgical Technique

The basic goal behind trabeculectomy is to create a small hole in the anterior chamber of the eye to allow drainage of the aqueous fluid toward the outside (Figure 8-5). Trabeculectomy surgery starts with making an incision through the conjunctiva. The surgeon then creates a partial-thickness *sclera flap* (or trapdoor) on the *sclera* (eye wall). Underneath the scleral flap, a surgeon cuts a small hole into the anterior chamber, which allows the drainage of aqueous fluid through the scleral flap and into the sub-conjunctival space. An *iridectomy* (hole in the iris) is performed at this point to allow the scleral opening to stay open without being blocked by the iris tissue. The scleral flap is then tied down with stitches that are loose enough to allow continuous drainage of the aqueous fluid. Finally, the overlying conjunctival tissue is closed with stitches to allow formation of a *bleb* or an elevation of conjunctival tissue formed by the aqueous fluid which is being filtered out of the scleral flap (trapdoor) underneath. The *filtering bleb* is usually located in the superior (upper) aspect of the eye and covered by the upper lid. Consequently, it is not readily noticeable by a casual observer. The aqueous fluid from the filtering bleb is then slowly absorbed by the conjunctival and episcleral (on the surface of the sclera) blood vessels and drain into the orbital venous system.

Starting in the late 1980's, chemotherapeutic drugs (or *anti-metabolite* or anti-healing medications commonly used in cancer chemotherapy) have been used during or after trabeculectomy. These anti-metabolite drugs are used to decrease the amount of tissue healing following trabeculectomy. A large multi-center study has shown that 5-fluorouracil (an anti-metabolite medication) is effective in increasing the success rate of trabeculectomy. Anti-metabolites such as 5-fluorouracil and mitomycin C are widely used during trabeculectomy to increase the overall success of the surgery. On the other hand, the frequent use of the anti-metabolite medications during trabeculectomy can also increase the risk of *hypotony* (low intraocular pressure *below* the physiologic level), which is one of the complications of trabeculectomy (see below).

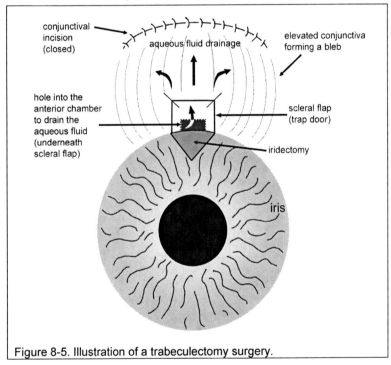

Figure 8-5. Illustration of a trabeculectomy surgery.

Postoperative Recovery and Follow-Up

Postoperatively, the recovery period is between 6-8 weeks. In trabeculectomy, the post-operative follow-up is particularly important because the success of the surgery depends on the rate and extent of conjunctival healing process. During this period, the surgeon follows

83

the patient closely, usually on a weekly (sometime more frequent) basis initially. During follow-up visits, adjustments can be made to reduce the intraocular pressure if it is too high. This can be done by cutting (or pulling) stitches from the scleral flap with a laser to allow additional filtration (*laser suture lysis,* Figure 8-6). If trabeculectomy is successful, it produces a nice *filtering bleb* (Figure 8-7), which is an elevation in conjunctival tissue indicating active filtration process underneath. Occasionally, the surgeon may elect to *needle the bleb* postoperatively if there is an excessive conjunctival scarring process. A small gauge needle is used to break up the scar tissue to allow more filtration of the aqueous fluid, and usually performed in a minor procedure room under topical anesthesia. If the intraocular pressure is too low, the surgeon may reduce the amount of anti-inflammatory (or steroid) medications to allow additional healing process. In short, there are many adjustments that may need to be done postoperatively to maximize the chance of surgical success. Thus, it is very important for the patient to have proper postoperative follow-up under the direction of the treating surgeon.

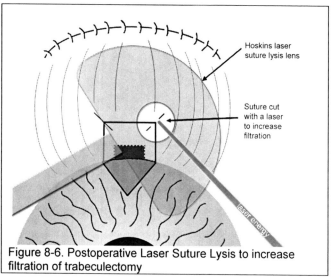

Hoskins laser
suture lysis lens

Suture cut
with a laser
to increase
filtration

laser energy

Figure 8-6. Postoperative Laser Suture Lysis to increase filtration of trabeculectomy

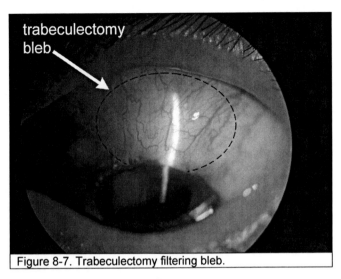

trabeculectomy
bleb

Figure 8-7. Trabeculectomy filtering bleb.

Success and Complications of Surgery

The success rate of a trabeculectomy is approximately 70-75%. Additional 10-15% can have a qualified success, meaning the goal intraocular pressure is achieved using one or more anti-glaucoma medication(s) postoperatively. Approximately 10-15% of the trabeculectomy may fail in the first year due to excessive conjunctival scarring. In approximately 1% of the time however, there can be more serious complications such as hemorrhage (bleeding), infection, and other complications. Depending on the complication, it may result in temporary or even permanent reduction in vision. It may also require further surgical procedure to correct the complication. It is important to discuss these potential complications with the treating physician before surgery.

The most common short-term *complication* of trabeculectomy surgery is that it may fail to adequately lower the intraocular pressure. This may occur due to the excessive scarring of the conjunctival tissue with decreased filtration of the aqueous fluid out of the eye. On the other hand, the intraocular pressure may be too low (called *hypotony*) due to the excessive filtering of the aqueous fluid or leaking wound. Low intraocular pressure (typically below 5 mmHg) can cause blurry vision and can be associated with shallowing of the anterior chamber, cataract formation, and greater risk of intraocular fluid accumulation (*choroidal effusion*) or *intraocular bleeding* (*suprachoroidal hemorrhage*). The suprachoroidal hemorrhage is a particularly feared complication after trabeculectomy, because it is often associated with pain, elevated intraocular pressure, and permanent decrease in vision. It often requires additional surgery to drain the blood.

There are also long-term complications of having a trabeculectomy bleb around the eye. If there is a leak from the bleb, the intraocular pressure may become too low. In addition, the bleb leak can increase the risk of infection. An infection in a post-trabeculectomy eye can be serious because of the surgical hole in the sclera may allow a direct access by the offending micro-organism to the inside of the eye. Such intraocular infection can seriously compromise the vision and even integrity of the eye itself. Therefore, any symptoms of infection in a post-trabeculectomy eye such as pain, decreased vision, redness, and purulent discharge, should be reported and examined promptly. This may occur even years after the surgery. For this reason, post-trabeculectomy patients are encouraged to always wear goggles during swimming and are discouraged from wearing contact lenses in order to decrease the possibility of a bleb infection (called *blebitis* or *bleb-associated endophthalmitis*).

Even a successful trabeculectomy surgery may not last forever; the surgery is considered successful if it controls the intraocular pressure for a period of 7-8 years. If the first trabeculectomy fails, it can be repeated to control glaucoma. Subsequent trabeculectomies usually have a higher chance of failure than the primary trabeculectomy surgery. If trabeculectomy fails to control glaucoma adequately, the surgeon may consider a glaucoma tube shunt (or *seton*) (see below).

8-C. Glaucoma Tube Shunt (Seton Implant)

A glaucoma drainage device or tube shunt is usually implanted when glaucoma is uncontrolled with medications, laser, or trabeculectomy. It is also used when there is not enough healthy tissue to proceed with trabeculectomy or in cases where trabeculectomy would likely fail. The goal of the glaucoma tube shunt is to allow aqueous fluid to leave the eye so that intraocular pressure will be lowered and halt the progression of glaucomatous visual loss.

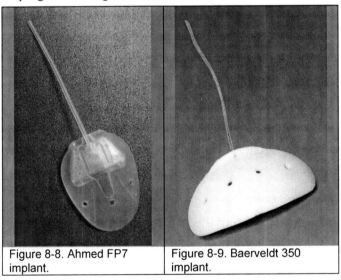

| Figure 8-8. Ahmed FP7 implant. | Figure 8-9. Baerveldt 350 implant. |

Several models of glaucoma tube shunts exist. The implants are typically made of silicone or polypropylene. Ahmed (Figure 8-8, New World Medical, Inc., Rancho Cucamonga, CA), Krupin (Hood Laboratories, Pembroke, MA), Baerveldt (Figure 8-9, Advanced

Medical Optics, Inc., Santa Ana, CA), and Molteno (IOP Inc., Costa Mesa, CA) tube shunts are the most common implants available. The glaucoma drainage devices are tubes, which are attached to a plate, and allow aqueous fluid to drain from the inside to outside of the eye. Both the tube and plate are covered by donor tissue and by patient's own conjunctiva. A glaucoma tube shunt can be with or without a valve. The tube shunts with a valve (Ahmed and Krupin) are made so that a set pressure is required before the tube opens and begins to drain aqueous fluid. They are usually implanted in cases where an immediate lowering of intraocular pressure is desired. The tube shunts without a valve (Baerveldt and Molteno) have no resistance to outflow of aqueous fluid, which may result in too low of an intraocular pressure (*hypotony*) initially. Severe or prolonged hypotony may lead to decreased vision or hemorrhage. To avoid these complications, the non-valved tube is often tied off with a dissolvable suture. The suture dissolves in approximately 6 weeks. During this time period, scar tissue develops over the tube plate which causes the required resistance to outflow that is necessary to avoid hypotony. Patients with non-valved tube shunts are forewarned that the vision may suddenly become blurry with floaters about 6 weeks after surgery when the tube opens. The symptoms typically resolve over time.

Indication for Tube Shunt Surgery

Drainage implant surgery is used in patients who may have failed other filtering surgeries and need a lower intraocular pressure. It is also useful in patients at higher risk of failure from trabeculectomy, due to previous scarring or inflammation of conjunctival tissue. Such conditions include neovascular glaucoma, uveitic (inflammatory) glaucoma, and conjunctival scarring from previous ocular surgeries. In these cases, glaucoma drainage device surgery may be more successful in controlling glaucoma.

The Tube Shunt Surgery

Prior to surgery, patients may be asked to stop any medication that "thins" the blood (e.g. aspirin, ibuprofen, warfarin, (Coumadin®), clopidogrel (Plavix®), or ticlopidine (Ticlid®)). Usually, this is coordinated with the primary care physician who is managing these medications. The surgery is typically performed under local anesthesia. Either a periocular injection of anesthetic is given, and/or topical medications to provide adequate pain control.

The conjunctiva in the designated quadrant of the eye is opened so that the eye muscles may be identified. The plate of the tube is placed between or underneath the eye muscles of the eye. It is fastened to the underlying sclera with permanent sutures. The tube is then cut to appropriate length and inserted into the anterior chamber. A small piece of donor tissue (sclera, cornea, pericardium, or dura) is then placed over the tube so that it does not erode through the overlying conjunctiva. The conjunctiva is placed back into place over the plate to cover the tube. In non-valved tubes, a dissolvable suture may be used to tie off the tube. The surgery is typically performed under local anesthesia in an outpatient setting.

Post-operative care

Patients who receive a valved implant are asked to discontinue their glaucoma medications after surgery, because the tube is expected to lower intraocular pressure immediately. During the postoperative course, glaucoma medications may be re-instituted based upon the level of intraocular pressure. Since non-valved implants do not work until approximately 6 weeks after surgery when the suture dissolves, patients are often asked to continue their glaucoma medications until this occurs. Once the tube opens and the intraocular pressure decreases, medications are discontinued as needed. In both types of tube shunt, patients are treated with topical steroids and antibiotics post-operatively. Occasionally pupil-dilating drops (*cycloplegics*) are used to keep the eye comfortable and to keep the anterior chamber well-formed.

Patients are asked to avoid heavy lifting, bending their head down below the waist, and getting dirty water in the eye. A shield is often used at night for eye protection initially. The postoperative visits are important since medication adjustments will be made after the intraocular pressure is checked. It is important not to dwell too much on the intraocular pressure in the early postoperative period since it can fluctuate significantly. It is not uncommon to have significant fluctuation in intraocular pressure during the first several weeks after glaucoma surgery.

Success Rates

In general, the success rate of glaucoma drainage devices is approximately 75% after 1-2 years. This varies slightly according to the type of tube shunt used and type of glaucoma being treated. Another 10-15% are successful with the addition of glaucoma medications (*partial success*). Failure to control intraocular pressure occurs in approximately 10%. These patients will need further surgical intervention to control their glaucoma.

Complications

Any ocular surgery including the glaucoma tube shunt has the potential complication of bleeding, infection, and discomfort. After tube shunt surgery, vision loss may occur from bleeding, infection, retinal detachment, swelling of the cornea or retina, hastening of cataract formation, or too low an eye pressure (*hypotony*). Additional glaucoma medications or surgery may be needed if the intraocular pressure remains higher than desired. The implant may also migrate or become exposed by eroding through the conjunctival tissue. Sometimes, the eyelid may become droopy (*ptosis*) after surgery or double vision (*diplopia*) may occur. These complications can be treated medically or surgically. Serious, vision-threatening complications are uncommon. If they occur, additional medication or surgery may be needed.

8-D. Ciliary body ablation (*cycloablation*)

When trabeculectomy or tube shunt has failed to control glaucoma, the treating physician may consider *cycloablation* (destruction of the ciliary body which produces the aqueous fluid). Because cycloablation involves permanent destruction of the ciliary body, it is usually the last line of treatment for uncontrolled glaucoma. Before the advent of laser, this was done using a *cryoprobe* (freezing probe) to freeze the ciliary body (*cyclocryotherapy*). This was often an uncomfortable procedure and was also associated with significant complications, including inflammation and loss of vision. Starting in the 1990's, *cyclocryotherapy* was largely replaced by a laser procedure called *CycloPhotoCoagulation* or CPC). At the University of Iowa, a portable diode laser is used to perform CPC under a local (retrobulbar) anesthesia in an outpatient setting (Figure 8-10). CPC usually takes less than 20 minutes to perform, including the anesthesia.

Cyclophotocoagulation (CPC) is a useful procedure for a refractive glaucoma which cannot be controlled by medications and other surgeries. The success rate for CPC is in the range of 60-70%, and it can be repeated if needed. The recovery period is usually 4-6 weeks. The follow up visits are not as intensive as the filtering surgery, and this may offer advantage to some patients. Post-operatively, the eye is treated with tapering regimen of anti-inflammatory steroids. There are a number of potential complications associated with *cyclophoto-coagulation (CPC)*, although less than those of cyclocryotherapy. Because CPC can be associated with a decrease in vision post-operatively, CPC is commonly reserved for patients who already have reduced vision from either glaucoma or other causes pre-operatively. CPC is also associated with increased inflammation, bleeding, and *hypotony* (low intraocular pressure (IOP) usually below 5 mmHg). Hypotony is feared complication of CPC because it is often difficult to raise the IOP after a permanent destruction of the ciliary body. Fortunately, it rarely occurs in CPC.

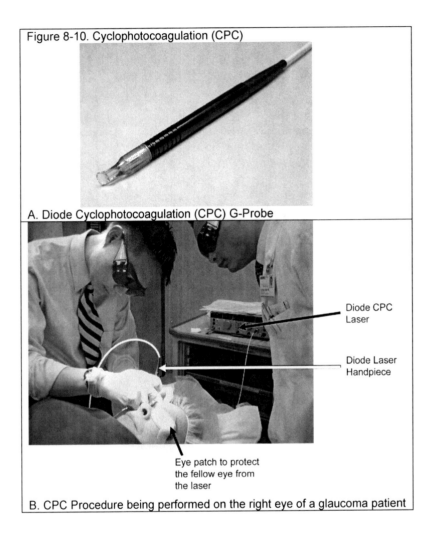

Figure 8-10. Cyclophotocoagulation (CPC)

A. Diode Cyclophotocoagulation (CPC) G-Probe

Diode CPC Laser

Diode Laser Handpiece

Eye patch to protect the fellow eye from the laser

B. CPC Procedure being performed on the right eye of a glaucoma patient

Chapter 9

Glaucoma Emergency:
Acute angle-closure glaucoma

9-A. Introduction to acute angle-closure glaucoma

Acute angle-closure glaucoma is a serious eye condition in which the drainage angle becomes obstructed and the aqueous humor cannot exit the eye. The iris and cornea become pressed together and consequently, aqueous fluid cannot get to the trabecular meshwork and exit the eye. The result is a rapid elevation of intraocular pressure (IOP) that causes a constellation of symptoms including decreased vision, seeing halos around bright objects, pain, and nausea. The intraocular pressure may become dangerously high and prompt treatment is necessary to prevent irreversible vision loss.

Table 9-1. Symptoms of acute angle-closure glaucoma.
Decreased vision
Seeing "halos"
Pain
Nausea

The most common form of angle-closure glaucoma involves blockage of the pupil by the lens (*pupillary block*) and occurs in eyes that have narrow drainage angles. Pupillary block occurs when the lens comes in close contact with the iris around the pupil and prevents aqueous fluid from moving through the pupil (Figure 9-1). Aqueous fluid collects behind the iris and causes it to bow forward and block aqueous fluid from reaching the trabecular meshwork and exiting the eye. This abnormal configuration of the iris prevents normal flow of aqueous fluid through the pupil to the trabecular meshwork and causes an acute rise in intraocular pressure.

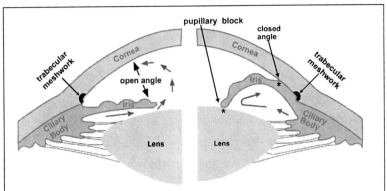

Figure 9-1. Acute angle-closure glaucoma.
Left: In an eye with a normal configuration of the anterior segment, the angle between the iris and cornea is wide open (approximately 40°). Aqueous fluid has free access to the trabecular meshwork and exits the eye unimpeded.
Right: In an eye with acute angle-closure, the angle between the iris and the cornea is obstructed and closed. Aqueous fluid is trapped behind iris and causes the iris to block trabecular meshwork resulting in rapid rise in intraocular pressure.

9-B. Risk Factors for acute angle-closure glaucoma

(also see Chapter 5-B)

There is variation in the size of the human eye. Some individuals have eyes that are smaller than the average. In such smaller eyes, there is relatively less space for the normal structures of the eye (ciliary body, lens, and iris) and consequently, these eyes have "crowded" drainage angles. The result is narrower drainage angles with less space between the lens and iris and a higher risk for pupillary block and acute closure of the drainage angle (Figure 9-1). The drainage angles of smaller eyes are therefore at higher risk of becoming critically narrow or closed. Consequently, acute angle-closure glaucoma occurs most commonly in people with traits that are associated with smaller eyes (Table 9-2).

Acute angle-closure glaucoma is more common in females because females have eyes that are generally smaller than those of males. Similarly, angle-closure glaucoma occurs more frequently with increasing age, because as the lens of the eye grows

Table 9-2. Risk factors for acute angle-closure glaucoma.
Female gender
Older age
Large natural lens (cataract)
Far-sightedness (Hyperopia)
Short axial length of the eye
Dim illumination
Certain Medications

larger with age, the anterior segment of the eye becomes more crowded and the drainage angle becomes narrower. People with eyes that are physically smaller are generally far-sighted (*hyperopic*) and require more corrective power for seeing nearby objects than distant objects. Such far-sighted (or hyperopic) individuals are at greater risk for acute angle-closure glaucoma, because the drainage angle in their smaller eyes is more crowded than in individuals with normal sized eyes. The risk for pupillary block and angle-closure is increased when the pupil is dilated by dim illumination or by medication. As the pupil gets bigger, the bulk of the iris moves towards the angle causing it to become more crowded and narrower. Dilation of the pupils can cause narrow angles to become abruptly closed in susceptible individuals.

When critically narrow angles are observed by an eye doctor, preventative laser surgery (laser peripheral iridotomy) is recommended to reduce the risk of angle-closure glaucoma occurring (see below).

9-C. Diagnosis of acute angle-closure glaucoma

Acute angle-closure glaucoma can be diagnosed with an examination by an eye doctor. Some of the common signs of acute angle-closure may be recognized by examination of the eye (Table 9-3).

Table 9-3. Signs of acute angle-closure glaucoma
Cloudy cornea Red eyes Forward bowing iris (from narrow or closed drainage angle) Mid-dilation of the pupil High intraocular pressure (several times higher than   normal pressure)

Pupillary block and obstruction of the drainage angle causes the iris to bow forward, which can be recognized with a slit lamp exam by an eye doctor (Figure 9-2). This abnormal configuration of the iris and cornea blocks outflow of fluid from the eye and causes the intraocular pressure to become rapidly elevated.

When the intraocular pressure (IOP) becomes very high, the "whites" of the eyes become red. High IOP also causes the normally clear cornea to become hazy which can decrease the vision. Changes in the cornea may also cause patients to see halos around bright objects. Finally, in acute angle-closure the pupil can be partially dilated and poorly responsive to light (Figure 9-3).

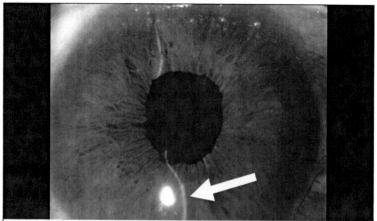

Figure 9-2. Abnormal forward bowing iris characteristic of acute angle-closure glaucoma. A key feature of acute angle-closure glaucoma is the abnormal forward position of the iris. When a straight beam of light is projected on an eye with acute angle-closure glaucoma, the beam (indicated by an arrow) appears curved due to the forward bowing of the iris.

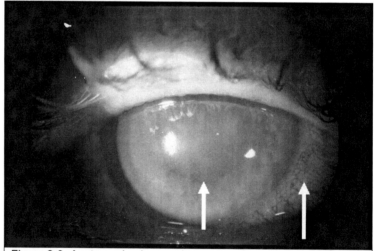

Figure 9-3. Acute angle-closure glaucoma, external appearance. Blockage of the drainage angle causes intraocular pressure to rise. High pressure results in a constellation of signs including redness of conjunctiva (right arrow), haziness of the cornea, and a mid-dilated pupil (left arrow).

Rapid elevation of intraocular pressure (IOP) is a key feature of acute angle-closure glaucoma. The pressure may rise as high as several times the normal IOP and can cause temporary or even permanent vision loss. Consequently, it is crucial to treat acute angle-closure glaucoma promptly.

9-D. Treatment of acute angle-closure glaucoma

Intraocular pressure may be critically high in acute angle-closure glaucoma. The goals of treatment are to lower the pressure as soon as possible and to prevent further attacks. Initially, acute angle-closure glaucoma is treated with a range of medicines that may be given as eye drops or pills. In rare cases intravenous medications may also be used. However, the definitive treatment for most cases of angle-closure glaucoma is laser peripheral iridotomy.

In most cases of angle-closure glaucoma, medications are used first to lower the eye pressure to a point at which the laser peripheral iridotomy (see Chapter 8-A(2)) can safely be performed. While medications may temporarily treat an episode of acute angle-closure, laser peripheral iridotomy is necessary to definitively treat and prevent future attacks. The treatments for acute angle-closure glaucoma are discussed in more detail below:

Topical medications

Most of the same eye-drops that are used for chronic forms of glaucoma (Chapter 7) are also used to treat acute angle-closure glaucoma. The combined use of several medications is generally required to sufficiently lower the intraocular pressure.

Three classes of medications reduce the production of aqueous fluid (beta blockers, alpha adrenergic agonists, and carbonic anhydrase inhibitors) and thereby lower pressure in the eye. These aqueous suppressant medications are useful in lowering the pressure in acute angle-closure glaucoma. Rapid application of a series of beta blockers, alpha adrenergic agonists, and carbonic anhydrase inhibitors eye drops will often lower intraocular pressure sufficiently to allow definitive treatment with a laser.

Once the eye pressure has been lowered with other medications, cholinergic eye drops may be used to pull the iris centrally in preparation for a laser treatment. The cholinergic eye drops stretch the iris and make it easier for the laser to produce a hole in the iris.

Oral medications

When topical eye-drops fail to lower intraocular pressure to safe levels, oral medications may be necessary in treating acute angle-closure glaucoma. Two forms of oral carbonic anhydrase inhibitors (acetazolamide and methazolamide) can be used to treat acute angle-closure glaucoma by reducing the production of aqueous fluid. Occasionally, a hyperosmotic drug (glycerol or isosorbide) may be used. The latter medications help to draw fluid out of the eye and into the bloodstream, thereby lowering the intraocular pressure.

Intravenous medications

Intravenous medications may rarely be necessary when topical and oral medications fail to adequately lower the intraocular pressure or when a patient is too sick to take oral medications. Intravenous hyperosmotic agents (urea or mannitol) may be used in these situations.

Laser treatment (Laser Peripheral Iridotomy)

A laser peripheral iridotomy to break the pupillary block and acute closure of the drainage angle should be performed as soon as possible after using medications. The goal of a laser peripheral iridotomy is to produce a hole in the iris to relieve the pupillary block and allow aqueous fluid to make its way to the trabecular meshwork, thereby lowering the intraocular pressure (Figure 9-4).

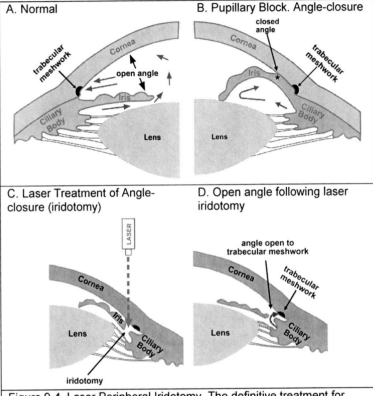

Figure 9-4. Laser Peripheral Iridotomy. The definitive treatment for acute angle-closure glaucoma is laser peripheral iridotomy.
A. Normal flow of aqueous humor in an eye with an open drainage angle.
B. In acute angle-closure glaucoma aqueous humor cannot pass through the pupil (pupillary block). Fluid collects behind the iris causing it to bow forward and close the drainage angle. The obstruction of aqueous humor drainage causes a rapid rise in intraocular pressure.
C. The treatment for acute angle-closure glaucoma using the laser to produce a hole in the iris (laser iridotomy).
D. Aqueous humor can bypass the pupil and make its way to the trabecular meshwork and out of the eye. Bypass of the pupillary block relieves bowing of the iris and opens the drainage angle.

The small hole in the iris created by laser peripheral iridotomy is not easily seen by the naked eye but can be recognized by an eye doctor during an exam (Figure 9-5).

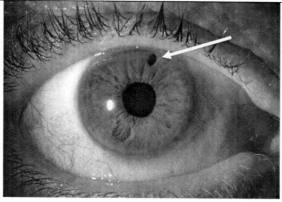

Figure 9-5. Laser peripheral iridotomy (LPI). The laser treatment for acute angle-closure glaucoma creates a small hole in the iris (arrow) that is visible with an eye examination.

9-E. Prevention

Before any attacks occur (prevention for both eyes)

Critically narrow drainage angles may be recognized prior to an attack of acute angle-closure. Such drainage angles may be identified by an eye doctor by gonioscopy (Chapter 6-C). When detected, critically narrow drainage angles need treatment with a laser peripheral iridotomy (see above) to prevent the attack of acute angle-closure glaucoma. In most cases laser peripheral iridotomy is performed in one eye at a time, within a few days to weeks of each other.

After an attack (prevention in the other eye)

When a patient has an attack of acute angle-closure glaucoma in one eye, it is treated emergently. In many cases, the fellow (uninvolved) eye also has a critically narrow drainage angle and is at high risk for acute angle-closure as well. A laser peripheral iridotomy should be performed to prevent acute angle-closure in the fellow eye as soon as the eye with acute angle-closure becomes stable after treatment.

Chapter 10

Pediatric Glaucoma

10-A. Types of pediatric glaucoma

Pediatric glaucoma (also referred to as *childhood glaucoma, infantile glaucoma* or *congenital glaucoma*) is a relatively rare disease, as most patients with glaucoma are adults. However, pediatric glaucoma can lead to loss of vision and blindness in a young child and will profoundly affect the child's life, if not diagnosed promptly and treated appropriately. Pediatric glaucoma can include a number of different diagnoses. *Primary congenital glaucoma* occurs in the first 3 years of life (usually within the first 6 months of life) without associated ocular or systemic abnormalities. Other pediatric glaucomas are associated with ocular and/or systemic abnormalities, or due to another disease (Table 10-1). The remainder of this chapter describes the primary congenital glaucoma.

The primary congenital glaucoma is thought to be an autosomal recessive disease and can be associated with a positive family history. However, in many cases of primary congenital glaucoma there is no obvious family history. It occurs approximately one in 30,000 live births, and the risk for congenital glaucoma is increased if there is a pre-existing family history. Molecular genetic studies have identified CYP1B1 gene as a cause for congenital glaucoma in patients with a positive family history (see Chapter 11).

Table 10-1. Different types of pediatric glaucomas.	
Primary pediatric glaucoma associated with ocular abnormalities	Aniridia
	Axenfeld-Rieger syndrome
	Congenital hereditary endothelial dystrophy (CHED)
	Congenital microcornea with myopia
	Congenital ocular melanosis (Nevus of Ota)
	Peters anomaly
	Posterior polymorphous dystrophy (PPMD)
	Sclerocornea
Primary pediatric glaucoma associated with systemic abnormalities	Axenfeld-Rieger syndrome
	Congenital rubella
	Cutis marmorata telangiectasia congenita
	Marfan syndrome
	Neurofibromatosis 1
	Oculocerebrorenal (Lowe) syndrome
	Stickler syndrome
	Sturge-Weber syndrome
Secondary pediatric glaucoma	Trauma
	Intraocular tumors (e.g., retinoblastoma)
	Uveitis (ocular inflammation)
	Lens-induced
	Aphakic (after cataract surgery without lens implant)
	Steroid-induced
	Ocular infection
	Angle-closure (e.g., retinopathy of prematurity)

10-B. Diagnosis of congenital glaucoma

Congenital glaucoma occurs in the first three years of life. Most commonly, patients are diagnosed between 3 and 6 months of age. In the United States, boys are slightly more commonly affected than girls. Approximately 70% of congenital glaucoma patients have both eyes affected, while the remaining 30% have only one eye affected.

There are three common symptoms associated with congenital glaucoma (Table 10-2). These include tearing (*epiphora*, Figure 10-1), light sensitivity (*photophobia*, Figure 10-2), and spasm and closure of the eyelids (*blepharospasm*, Figure 10-2) due to the patient's sensitivity to light.

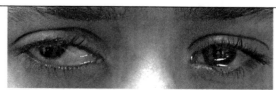

Figure 10-1. Light sensitivity and tearing in a teenage patient with a long history of congenital glaucoma. He also has misalignment of the eyes (*strabismus*).

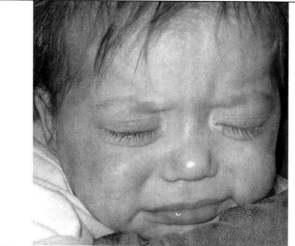

Figure 10-2. Spasm and closure of the eyelids (*blepharospasm*) and light sensitivity (*photophobia*) of a patient with congenital glaucoma.

On eye examination, there are certain features that are commonly associated with congenital glaucoma (Table 10-2). Patients often avoid bright lights because they are very sensitive to light. This is from the cloudy, hazy cornea that disperses the light and causes glare.

Instead of a normally clear cornea, these patients develop a thick, cloudy, and hazy cornea (frosted glass appearance) from elevated intraocular pressure (IOP). In severe cases, the patient's pupil may not even be visible due to the cloudy cornea. Over time, the elevated IOP can cause "stretch marks" in the cornea from excessive stretching (*Haab's striae*, Figure 10-3), and also enlarge the size of the eye itself (*buphthalmos*, Figure 10-4).

Table 10-2. Common symptoms and signs of primary congenital glaucoma	
Symptoms	Tearing (*epiphora*)
	Light sensitivity (*photophobia)*
	Spasm and closure of eyelids (*blepharospasm*)
Signs	Elevated intraocular pressure (IOP)
	Enlarged cornea
	Cloudy, hazy cornea (*corneal edema*)
	Tears in Descemet's membrane in cornea (*Haab's striae*)
	Enlarged length of the eye (*buphthalmos*)
	Optic nerve damage (cupping)

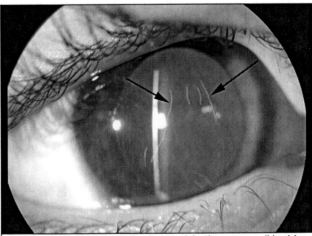

Figure 10-3. Stretch marks (arrows) in the cornea (Haab's striae) from the high intraocular pressure in a patient with congenital glaucoma.

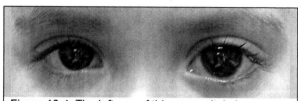

Figure 10-4. The left eye of this congenital glaucoma patient is noticeably larger than the right eye. The patient has buphthalmos of the left eye.

Abnormal enlargement of one or both eyes in an infant is an important sign of congenital glaucoma and should not be ignored. Eventually, as in adult glaucoma, the optic nerve will become damaged with cupping (see Chapter 1). Unlike adult glaucoma, the optic nerve damage in congenital glaucoma can be reversible in the early stages if the glaucoma is treated promptly and effectively.

10-C. Treatment of congenital glaucoma

Unlike adult glaucoma, the initial treatment for congenital glaucoma is often surgical. A "drainage angle surgery" is often recommended for congenital glaucoma. The most common surgical procedures for congenital glaucoma are goniotomy and trabeculotomy. While they are considered to have similar rates of success (80-90%), some surgeons prefer one technique over the other. One advantage of trabeculotomy over goniotomy is that a clear cornea is not necessary to perform the procedure, while a reasonably clear cornea is necessary for goniotomy. The goniotomy surgery involves entering the anterior chamber with a sharp goniotomy knife and making an opening incision through the abnormally developed trabecular meshwork . This allows greater outflow of the aqueous fluid and thereby, lower the intraocular pressure (Figure 10-5). Often 100-120 degrees (out of 360 degrees total) of the trabecular meshwork can be treated with goniotomy in a single setting. Trabeculotomy surgery involves making an external incision and identifying the Schlemm's canal from the outside, inserting a fine instrument into the Schlemm's canal, and breaking through the trabecular meshwork to increase the aqueous outflow (Figure 10-6). Typically, 120-140 degrees of trabecular meshwork can be treated by trabeculotomy in a single surgery. If one surgical technique is unsuccessful in decreasing the intraocular pressure, the other technique can be utilized in a fresh area of the trabecular meshwork (the area not previously operated upon) to increase the success of the surgery. Even after initial control of the intraocular pressure is established with surgery, a periodic monitoring is necessary to ensure the intraocular pressure doesn't increase again and the glaucoma go out of control.

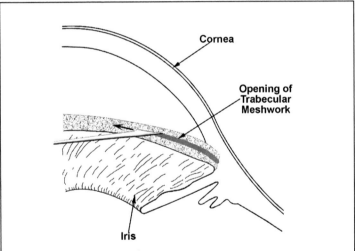

Figure 10-5. Goniotomy. A fine surgical knife is used to open the drainage angle (trabecular meshwork) in order to lower the intraocular pressure.

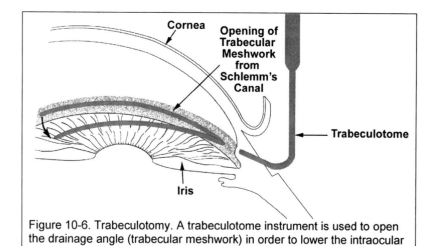

Figure 10-6. Trabeculotomy. A trabeculotome instrument is used to open the drainage angle (trabecular meshwork) in order to lower the intraocular pressure.

Medications can be used as an adjunct therapy either before or after the surgical treatment. Medications may be utilized temporarily after the diagnosis until surgery can be performed. If the initial surgery fails to completely control the intraocular pressure, topical medications can be used to bring the glaucoma under control. The systemic side effects of topical medications are greater in infants than in adults because of the smaller body mass. Because of potential systemic side effects, the first line of medications that are commonly employed is the topical carbonic anhydrase inhibitors (CAI, see Chapter 7). After the CAI, the next choices are topical prostaglandin analogs or beta-blockers (Chapter 7). The prostaglandin analogs appear to be safe in children; however, there are no long-term data on the safety of these medications in children. Topical beta-blockers should be used with caution in children because of the well-known systemic side effects (Chapter 7). Finally, topical alpha-2 agonist (brimonidine, Chapter 7) should be *avoided* in infants because it's been associated with severe respiratory depression (breathing difficulty).

10-D. Importance of team approach in pediatric glaucoma

It takes a whole team of physicians, nurses, and family to provide an optimal treatment for patients with pediatric glaucoma. For example, a glaucoma specialist may provide care for pediatric glaucoma, while a pediatric ophthalmologist may simultaneously treat a "lazy eye" (*amblyopia*). Lazy eye is a condition in which the visual part of the child's brain does not develop properly due to abnormalities of the eye (for example, glaucoma) or eye alignment (*strabismus*). Pediatric glaucoma patients are at a high risk for development of amblyopia, unless they are closely monitored and treated. If amblyopia is detected, the child needs to be promptly treated because the amblyopia becomes irreversible and not amenable to treatment after the age of approximately 10 years.

It is critical to have a total commitment of the family as well. The family is asked to bring the patient to multiple doctors over many months or years for the treatment of glaucoma. The child may undergo multiple sedations or anesthesia, just to check the intraocular pressure and perform adequate ocular examination. The family is often asked to administer multiple eye drops every day as part of the glaucoma treatment. All of these activities can add a significant amount of stress to the family as well as the patient. On the other hand, when everyone works together to provide an optimal treatment, there is a reasonable chance that the child with glaucoma can grow up with good eyesight.

Chapter 11

Genetics of glaucoma

Heredity plays an important role in most forms of glaucoma. In some types of glaucoma, such as in juvenile open-angle glaucoma, disease clearly runs in families. On the other hand, the contribution of genetic factors to other types of glaucoma, such as primary open-angle glaucoma, may be less obvious. Many genetic factors that are involved in the development of glaucoma are discussed in more detail below.

11-A. Genetic basis of glaucoma

Several lines of evidence indicate that glaucoma has a genetic basis, that is, glaucoma is caused in part by defects in specific genes (Table 11-1). First, although many cases of glaucoma occur with no family history of disease, glaucoma appears to be clearly heritable in some families. A number of large families have been reported in which glaucoma is inherited as a simple Mendelian trait (usually with autosomal dominant inheritance). Studies of the epidemiology of glaucoma also support the notion that there is a significant genetic component. Relatives of individuals affected with glaucoma have a higher risk of developing glaucoma when compared to the general population. Additionally, many of the individual signs of glaucoma are heritable themselves, including cup-to-disc ratio and intraocular pressure. When these key features of glaucoma are examined individually, they appear to run in families. Lastly, the frequency of glaucoma varies greatly between different ethnic and racial groups. For example, the prevalence of glaucoma in blacks is significantly higher than that of whites, which suggests that blacks have a higher risk of developing glaucoma due to a heritable factor that is more prevalent in this racial group.

Table 11-1. Evidence that glaucoma is caused at least in part by genes.
Families that show clear inheritance of glaucoma
Relatives of glaucoma patients have a higher rate of developing glaucoma themselves
Features of glaucoma (large cup-to-disc ratio and high intraocular pressure) are heritable
Glaucoma is more common in some ethnic and racial groups than others

11-B. Research methods for studying glaucoma genetics

Two general approaches to study the genetics of glaucoma are candidate gene screening and positional cloning. The advantages of each of these types of investigations are discussed below.

Candidate gene approach to glaucoma

The core features of the candidate gene approach are: 1) making a list of *candidate* genes that might cause glaucoma if their normal function is altered and 2) testing a large group of unrelated glaucoma patients for defects in these candidate genes.

Identifying candidate genes.

Several types of genes are suspected of having a role in the development of glaucoma. Some of the best candidate genes have functions that suggest they may be important in glaucoma such as (1) genes that are active in the drainage angle where fluid leaves the eye; (2) genes that are active in the ciliary body where fluid is made in the eye; (3) genes with functions that suggest they regulate the intraocular pressure; and 4) genes that may be important in maintaining the health of the optic nerve.

Testing candidate genes.

Candidate genes are evaluated for a possible role in causing glaucoma by testing the DNA of large numbers of unrelated glaucoma patients for disease-causing defects. Candidate gene screening is a useful research approach to discover disease-causing genes. This research is dependent on the enrollment of hundreds of volunteer subjects with glaucoma. By participating in candidate gene studies of glaucoma, patients may learn something about the reasons why they developed glaucoma as well as help with research efforts to study the disease.

Positional cloning approach to glaucoma (linkage analysis).

Linkage analysis is a method for identifying glaucoma-causing genes that is dependent solely on the availability of large families with several members that have glaucoma. DNA is collected from each member of these families and is tested to see which segments of the DNA are always passed down through the family along with glaucoma. Genes that cause glaucoma are located within these *linked* regions of DNA (Figure 11-1).

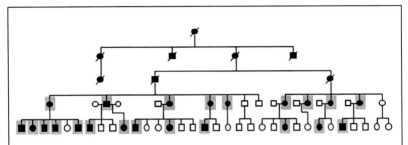

Figure 11-1. Linkage Analysis of Glaucoma. This diagram represents the family tree of a family affected with glaucoma. The males in the family are represented by squares and the females are represented by circles. Deceased family members have a diagonal line across the symbol. Family members affected with glaucoma are indicated by shading the pedigree symbols black. Most spouses were omitted from the diagram. In linkage analysis the inheritance of genetic markers (represented in the diagrams of a family tree with darkened squares) is compared to inheritance of glaucoma (represented by darkly shaded pedigree symbols). The inheritance of a genetic marker on chromosome 1 is represented by the shaded boxes. Notice that the shaded boxes are always passed down through the family together with glaucoma. Therefore the gene causing glaucoma in this family is located near this genetic marker on chromosome 1.

Linkage analysis identifies where glaucoma genes are located within the genome. The next step is testing members of the family for disease-causing defects in the genes that are located with the linked regions.

Linkage analysis has some advantages that make it particularly well-suited for searching for glaucoma genes. This approach to finding disease-causing genes is possible even when little is known about the basic biological mechanisms of the disease being studied (such as glaucoma). This research is dependent on the identification and enrollment of large families with many members that are affected with glaucoma. Most of the known glaucoma genes were discovered with linkage analysis of large glaucoma families.

11-C. The genetics of specific types of glaucoma

Several forms of glaucoma have been investigated in search of disease-causing genes. In recent years, genes associated with juvenile open-angle glaucoma, primary open-angle glaucoma, primary congenital glaucoma, and many forms of secondary glaucoma have been identified (Table 11-2). The genes associated with juvenile open-angle glaucoma, normal tension glaucoma, and primary congenital glaucoma are reviewed below.

Table 11-2. Known glaucoma-causing genes. Several genes have been associated with various forms of glaucoma including juvenile open-angle glaucoma (JOAG), primary open-angle glaucoma (POAG), primary congenital glaucoma (PCG), Axenfeld-Rieger's syndrome (ARS), anterior segment dysgenesis syndrome (ASD), and aniridia.

Gene	Chromosomal location	Type of Glaucoma
Myocilin (MYOC)	Chromosome 1q24.3-q25.2	JOAG or POAG
Optineurin (OPTN)	Chromosome 10p15-p14	NTG
Cytochrome P450 1B1 (CYP1B1)	Chromosome 2p22-p21	PCG
Paired homeodomain transcription factor 2 (PITX2)	Chromosome 4q25-q26	Glaucoma associated with ARS
Forkhead Box C1 (FOXC1)	Chromosome 6p25	Glaucoma associated with ASD and ARS
Paired box 6 (PAX6)	Chromosome 11p13	Glaucoma associated with aniridia

Juvenile open-angle glaucoma

Juvenile open-angle glaucoma (JOAG) is a rare form of glaucoma that accounts for approximately 1% of total glaucoma patients. The clinical features of JOAG are the same as those of more common forms of glaucoma (such as primary open-angle glaucoma). JOAG

116

differs from primary open-angle glaucoma (POAG) mainly in the severity of disease and age of onset. Patients with JOAG develop disease at a much earlier age (between 3 and 39 years) than patients with POAG. JOAG patients also have very high intraocular pressures that frequently exceed 40 mm Hg in the absence of treatment.

In many cases, JOAG clearly runs in families as a dominant trait. Due to the early age of onset and the strong clinical signs of JOAG, several large pedigrees with many generations of affected family members have been recognized (Figure 11-2).

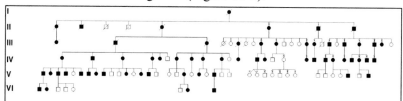

Figure 11-2. Juvenile open-angle glaucoma (JOAG) pedigree. JOAG is an early-onset form of open-angle glaucoma that is inherited as an autosomal dominant trait. Offspring of a parent with JOAG have up to a 50% chance of inheriting JOAG. This diagram shows the pattern of inheritance of glaucoma through an actual JOAG pedigree.

Genetic studies of large families (like the one shown in Figure 11-2) demonstrated that defects or mutations in the myocilin gene are a cause of JOAG. Most cases of JOAG that have a strong family history of disease are associated with defects in the myocilin gene (*MYOC*). Myocilin associated glaucoma is inherited as an autosomal dominant trait. That is, patients carrying a myocilin mutation that causes JOAG have a 50% chance of passing the gene (and high risk for glaucoma) to their children. Several specific defects or mutations in the myocilin gene that cause JOAG have been identified. Some patients have the typical clinical features of JOAG but do not have a family history of disease. The myocilin gene has a less important role in these sporadic cases of JOAG.

The myocilin gene directs tissues of the eye to produce a protein that is released into the aqueous humor. The myocilin protein has an unknown function; however, glaucoma develops when its structure is altered by a gene mutation. Studies are underway to investigate role of the myocilin gene in healthy eyes and the process by which defects in this gene lead to glaucoma.

Primary open-angle glaucoma

Primary open-angle glaucoma (POAG) is the most common form of glaucoma in the United States. Like juvenile onset open-angle glaucoma (JOAG), there is also a genetic basis to POAG. However, there are important differences between the genetics of POAG and JOAG. POAG runs in families, but the pattern of inheritance is more difficult to recognize. Due to the relatively late onset of disease in POAG (after the age of 40), most of the families with this condition only include one or two generations of affected family members that are alive. Parents of affected family members are often deceased and offspring of affected members are frequently too young to show signs of the disease. Consequently, families with inherited forms of POAG are generally small with only a few affected members and are difficult to distinguish from sporadic (non-familial) cases (Figure 11-3).

Although research has indicated that primary open-angle glaucoma (POAG) is heritable, most of the genes that cause this disease have not yet been identified. It is likely that some cases of POAG will be due to defects in a single gene, while other cases will be due to the combined effects of mutations in several genes and other environmental factors.

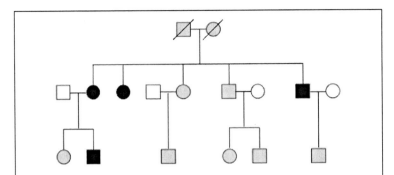

Figure 11-3 Primary Open-Angle Glaucoma (POAG) pedigree. This diagram shows an example of the pattern of inheritance of glaucoma that may occur in a POAG pedigree. The squares represent male family members, while the circles represent female family members. Darkly shaded symbols indicate an affected family member, while unshaded symbols indicate an unaffected family member. Grey symbols indicate a family member with unknown glaucoma status. Diagonal lines (through a square or circle) indicate that a particular family member is deceased. Notice that the founders of the family are deceased and it is unknown whether they were affected with POAG (indicated by grey boxes). Similarly, most of the grandchildren of the founders are younger than the age at which most people develop glaucoma. It is unknown whether these family members will later develop glaucoma so they are shaded grey to indicate their unknown glaucoma status. The majority of family members affected with POAG are in a single generation.

The identification of disease-causing genes has been an active focus of research studies of POAG. The approximate position in the genome, or locus, of many genes that can cause POAG has been determined by linkage analysis (Table 11-3). Loci for genes that cause POAG are designated by a code beginning with the letters "GLC1" and ending in a suffix letter for each new glaucoma loci in chronologic order of discovery. For example, GLC1A was the first open-angle glaucoma locus to be discovered. The glaucoma genes in two of these loci have been discovered (myocilin at the GLC1A locus and optineurin at the GLC1E locus). Research to find the disease-causing genes at the other loci is ongoing.

119

Table 11-3. Known loci (chromosome location) for primary forms of glaucoma. The chromosomal locations of 13 genes that cause glaucoma have been discovered. The type of glaucoma associated with each loci is indicated: Primary open-angle glaucoma (POAG), juvenile-onset open-angle glaucoma (JOAG), normal tension glaucoma (NTG), or primary congenital glaucoma (PCG). The disease-causing gene at three of these loci are known, while the remaining ten are as yet undiscovered.

Chromosomal Loci	Locus Name	Known Gene	Glaucoma
Chromosome 1q	GLC1A	*MYOC*	JOAG, POAG
Chromosome 2q	GLC1B	-	POAG
Chromosome 3q	GLC1C	-	POAG
Chromosome 8q	GLC1D	-	POAG
Chromosome 10p	GLC1E	*OPTN*	NTG
Chromosome 7q	GLC1F	-	POAG
Chromosome 5q	GLC1G	-	POAG
Chromosome 2p	GLC1H	-	POAG
Chromosome 15q	GLC1I	-	POAG
Chromosome 9q	GLC1J	-	POAG
Chromosome 20p	GLC1K	-	POAG
Chromosome 2p	GLC3A	*CYP1B1*	PCG
Chromosome 1p	GLC3B	-	PCG

At present, only one gene that causes primary open-angle glaucoma has been discovered (the myocilin gene at the GLC1A locus). As discussed above, one set of mutations in the myocilin gene are known to cause early onset glaucoma (juvenile open-angle glaucoma). A different set of mutations in the same myocilin gene can cause primary open-angle glaucoma. In fact mutations in the myocilin gene have been shown to be responsible for approximately 3-4% of worldwide cases of primary open-angle glaucoma. Myocilin associated glaucoma is inherited as an autosomal dominant trait and offspring of affected parents have a 50% chance of inheriting an abnormal myocilin gene, which confers a high risk for developing glaucoma.

Myocilin defects have been identified in patients with primary open-angle glaucoma from different races and ethnicities including Caucasians from Midwestern United States; Caucasians from Canada; Caucasians from Australia; African Americans from New York City; and Asians from Gifu, Japan. In all populations approximately 1 in 25 cases of primary open-angle glaucoma are due to abnormalities of the myocilin gene. One set of defects in the myocilin gene cause juvenile open-angle glaucoma while a different set of defects cause primary open-angle glaucoma. In many cases, when a particular defect in the myocilin gene is detected, the severity of the associated glaucoma (age of onset and maximum intraocular pressure) can be predicted.

Myocilin mutations account for approximately 3-4% of cases of primary open-angle glaucoma. It is likely that many additional genes are involved in the development of glaucoma. The search for these genes is an area of ongoing research.

Normal tension glaucoma.

Most cases of normal tension glaucoma (NTG) are sporadic with no clear family history. However, rare cases of families with many affected members have been reported. In these families, normal tension glaucoma (NTG) is inherited as an autosomal dominant trait. Genetic studies have shown that mutations in a gene known as *optineurin* (*OPTN*) are responsible for a significant fraction of familial NTG cases. A single optineurin mutation has been associated with glaucoma in several large NTG families. The role of the optineurin gene in sporadic cases of NTG has not been clearly defined.

More is known about the optineurin gene than the myocilin gene. The optineurin gene produces a protein that appears to have many functions. Some studies suggest that optineurin is involved in *apoptosis*, which is a process by which cells self-destruct or "commit suicide". It is possible that the optineurin gene may cause optic nerve damage and glaucoma by promoting apoptosis of this tissue. Current studies are exploring the precise mechanism by which defects in the optineurin gene lead to glaucoma.

Primary congenital glaucoma (PCG)

Many cases of primary congenital glaucoma appear to be sporadic; however, as many as 10-40% cases are familial with autosomal recessive inheritance. Many large primary congenital glaucoma pedigrees with clear autosomal recessive inheritance have been reported. In addition, twin studies have provided strong evidence that primary congenital glaucoma has a genetic basis. Twins with identical DNA (identical, monozygotic twins) tend to both have primary congenital glaucoma at a much higher rate than twins with only 50% identical DNA (fraternal, dizygotic twins). This difference in concordance indicates that genes have important roles in the development of primary congenital glaucoma.

Research studies of several large families have shown that mutations in the gene *cytochrome P450 1B1* (*CYP1B1*) cause many cases of primary congenital glaucoma. Most patients with primary congenital glaucoma (87% of familial cases and 27% of sporadic cases) have glaucoma due to variations in the CYP1B1 gene.

The CYP1B1 gene encodes a protein that metabolizes or breaks down certain molecules or drugs. The mechanism by which defects in the CYP1B1 gene causes primary congenital glaucoma is unknown. However, it has been theorized that mutations in this gene may alter its ability to break down factors that are vital to the normal development of drainage angle. A defective CYP1B1 gene might, therefore, result in an abnormal concentration of these developmental factors and lead to the abnormal formation of the drainage angle and primary congenital glaucoma.

11-D. Genetic testing for glaucoma

Spectacular progress in being made in the field of genetic research and important discoveries and innovations are being made at an increasingly rapid pace. In the last few years, several landmark discoveries have been made in ophthalmic genetics. *The Online Mendelian Inheritance in Man* (OMIM, www.ncbi.nlm.nih.gov) is a catalog of heritable diseases and syndromes. At the beginning of 2007, this database had 813 entries of heritable conditions that affect the eye and 171 conditions in which glaucoma is a feature. As new genes that cause various types of glaucoma are discovered, there will be more opportunities for genetic testing to enhance all aspects of patient care including diagnosis, prognosis, treatment, and family planning. Currently, genetic testing is available for several glaucoma genes including myocilin (*MYOC*), optineurin (*OPTN*), and cytochrome P450 1B1 (CYP1B1).

Genetic testing may be useful for patients with specific types of glaucoma and particular clinical features of the disease. Patients that are interested in testing should discuss it with their physician and/or a genetic counselor. Along with discussing whether genetic testing is appropriate for a particular type of glaucoma, physicians and counselors may discuss the implications of these investigations. Genetic testing for inherited diseases may provide information that is useful for a patient's medical care; however, this information may also affect other family members. Consequently, it is possible that genetic testing may be a source of stress or anxiety for the patient and for family members. Additionally, the results of genetic tests are complex, and should be interpreted by experienced physicians and genetic counselors. The meaning of positive or negative results is not always obvious, and must be carefully explained for genetic testing to be helpful to the patient. For example, there are likely many more glaucoma-causing genes than what have been discovered so far. If a patient is tested for defects in the known glaucoma genes (i.e. myocilin and optineurin) and no disease-causing mutations are detected, it is still possible that the patient developed glaucoma due to defects in other genes that have not yet been discovered. A patient's physician or counselor is best equipped to explain the meaning and consequences of such genetic test results.

Some general guidelines for who may benefit most from some specific types of genetic testing are provided below.

Myocilin genetic testing for Juvenile Open-Angle Glaucoma.

The patients with the highest likelihood of having glaucoma that is associated with a defect in the myocilin gene are patients with an early onset of disease (3 to 39 years of age); extremely high intraocular pressure (> 30 mm Hg); and a strong family history of disease. Most patients with these characteristics have familial juvenile-onset primary open-angle glaucoma that is due to a mutation in the myocilin gene. Genetic testing may provide patients with familial JOAG and their physicians useful information to help solidify a diagnosis of this form of glaucoma.

Myocilin (MYOC) genetic testing for Primary Open-Angle Glaucoma.

Mutations in the myocilin gene account for a smaller proportion of primary open-angle glaucoma (POAG) cases (3-4%) than JOAG. At present, due to the relatively low prevalence of myocilin-associated POAG and the labor-intensive nature of the mutation detection tests, large-scale testing of the general population for myocilin defects is not feasible. However, testing those individuals who are at extremely high risk for developing myocilin-associated POAG may be warranted. Such patients would include family members of patients with known myocilin-associated glaucoma and members of families with a strong history of inherited POAG.

Optineurin (OPTN) genetic testing for Normal Tension Glaucoma.

Most cases of normal tension glaucoma occur sporadically, without a family history of disease. However, there are rare familial cases of NTG and testing these patients for mutations in the optineurin gene may be warranted.

Cytochrome P450 1B1 (CYP1B1) testing for PCG.

Many cases of PCG are due to mutations in the *CYP1B1* gene. In certain European populations of patients, as much as 87% of family cases of PCG and 27% of sporadic cases of PCG are caused by mutations of the *CYP1B1* gene. However, the frequency of *CYP1B1* mutations in cases of PCG in the United States is not precisely known. Based on this information, it is usually reasonable to test for *CYP1B1* mutations in PCG patients with a positive family history of disease. While the likelihood of detecting a *CYP1B1* mutation in a PCG patient is lower when there is no family history of disease, genetic testing may be warranted in some of these sporadic cases.

11-E. Benefits of studying glaucoma genetics

Every year, thousands of Americans are blinded by glaucoma. In most cases, the loss of vision caused by glaucoma could be limited or prevented by currently available therapies if the disease were identified in its early stages. Many cases of glaucoma are not discovered until vision has already been permanently lost, because clinical signs of early glaucoma are subtle and silent to the patient.

The discovery of glaucoma disease genes provides a method for early detection of glaucoma. Genetic testing for disease-causing mutations in these genes is capable of identifying those at highest risk for developing glaucoma, perhaps years to decades before vision loss or other symptoms are manifested. Heightened surveillance and early institution of glaucoma therapy can then be provided to these patients before any vision is lost, even before any symptoms are observed.

Testing to determine the genetic causes of glaucoma will also facilitate the development and evaluation of new medical therapies and surgical interventions.

Glaucoma is a collection of distinct diseases with similar clinical appearances. Genetic testing will allow physicians to identify groups of patients with the same biochemical basis of glaucoma. Some subtypes of glaucoma may respond to certain treatments while others may not. Identification of such well-characterized groups of patients to test new medical therapies and surgical interventions will help speed the discovery of new, effective treatments.

Genetic study of inherited diseases such as glaucoma will likely promote advances in therapy as well as diagnosis. For example, methods to replace defective genes with normal functioning genes (trans-genes) are being studied. At present, however, there are limitations to this technology known as *gene therapy*. Some of the major obstacles in using gene therapy include difficulties in obtaining 1) effective delivery of the trans-genes to the right tissues of the eye, 2) control of transgene activity, 3) maintenance of transgene effect, and 4) low-cost methodology. Advances in all of these areas are being realized, and gene therapy for glaucoma may be possible in the future.

Most inherited genetic defects that cause glaucoma, however, may be treated with currently available medical and surgical therapies. As the functions of disease-causing genes are discovered, conventional treatments may also be tailored to mitigate disease-causing defects. There are many ways that genetic research opens the promise of a new generation of sight-saving therapies.

Chapter 12

12-A. Using Glaucoma Medications Regularly

The Patient-Doctor Relationship

The most important controllable factor in glaucoma management is adherence to prescribed medications. A good patient-doctor relationship fosters knowledge of the disease process and greater likelihood of adhering with a recommended regimen. The more patients know about their disease process, the more likely they are to adhere to treatment. A common misconception is that blindness is the inevitable result of glaucoma. While there is a possibility of blindness in glaucoma, it is not necessarily inevitable. With proper diagnosis and early intervention, most patients retain functional vision with limited visual disability. Asking questions and better understanding of the disease are part of effective treatment.

Understanding Goals of Treatment

Since glaucoma is a chronic condition, once treatment is initiated it is often continued for an extended period of time. The goal of medications is to prevent a further decline of vision by lowering the intraocular pressure (IOP). This goal is sometimes not obvious to patients because instead of restoring lost vision, it aims toward preventing further vision loss. The presumed lack of direct benefit hinders adherence with glaucoma medications. When there is no immediate benefit from taking medications, patients may be less inclined to take them as prescribed. In addition, the vision loss from glaucoma tends to occur slowly over time and there are usually no acute symptoms. Patients do not notice the vision loss that occurs over a long time period and fail to see this as being a result of not taking their glaucoma medications. Although the immediate benefit is not obvious, it is important to realize that taking daily eye drops decreases the likelihood of vision loss from glaucoma.

Worsening Glaucoma with Missed Doses

Missed doses of medications can cause vision loss, just as not taking glaucoma medications can. The fluctuations in intraocular pressure (IOP) can be detrimental to the optic nerve. A study which used electronically monitored medication bottles revealed that only 83% of timolol doses were taken as prescribed. The IOP measured the day of the exam can be misleading since most patients take their eye medications shortly prior to the examination. Unfortunately, there is no available physiologic parameter which allows the eye doctor to know what the average IOP has been between visits. Glaucoma can worsen when doses are repeatedly missed despite a good measurement at the doctor's office. It is important to realize that fluctuations of IOP, as well as high IOP, can be detrimental to the optic nerve.

A Team Approach to Battling Glaucoma

The treatment of glaucoma is a battle which must be fought by both the patient and eye doctor. It is very difficult, if not impossible, for an eye doctor to control glaucoma without the full participation of the patient. It is the patient who is responsible for the day-to-day treatment of glaucoma. The patient should be aware of the benefits and side effects of the recommended medications. A well-informed patient is more likely to adhere to a long-term medical treatment of glaucoma.

12-B. Adherence to Glaucoma Medication

Many studies have tried to evaluate the level of adherence in patients and the risk factors for nonadherence. In general, 13.4% to 60% of patients have reported their non-adherence when asked. Numerous factors have been evaluated to determine what affects adherence. Age, race, and gender have not been found to be contributing factors. Some of the contributory factors are discussed below.

12-B(1). Factors Affecting Adherence

Forgetfulness or Physical Limitations. Many patients report forgetfulness as one of the major reasons that they are not 100% adherent with their glaucoma medications. It is often difficult to incorporate a new drug regimen into one's lifestyle.

Physical Limitations. Those with physical limitations, such as severe arthritis or significant visual disability, may have problems self-administering medications. Family or caregivers can help treat glaucoma by accompanying the patient to appointments, understanding the disease, and learning how to administer eye drops if necessary.

Misunderstanding the Disease and Its Treatment. This factor is easily corrected by gathering information about the disease process. Information on glaucoma is readily available at your eye doctor's office, the library, book stores, and the internet (including the website for the online version of this book, www.medrounds.org/glaucoma-guide). These available resources are inexpensive and easily obtained.

Multiple Doses per Day. The number of doses per day and number of medications can also affect adherence. The more doses or medications prescribed, the less likely that there will be perfect adherence. Instilling numerous doses or medications can adversely affect a patient's lifestyle. It is difficult to remember to administer multiple eye drops throughout the day. The more frequently the dose, the more likely there will be missed doses. Given the time necessary to ensure proper glaucoma medications, it is easy to see why patients prefer once daily-dosed eye drops. The following eye drops are administered once daily: Xalatan®, Travatan®, Lumigan®, Timoptic XE®, Istalol®.

Multiple Medications. One can improve adherence by minimizing the dosage and total number of medications that are still effective. Patients should be on the least number of eye drops necessary with the least dosing per day to control their glaucoma. Written instructions from the doctor's office are a good reminder to be used at home, particularly for those on multiple systemic medications for other diseases. Combination eye drops [e.g., Cosopt® (timolol/dorzolamide) and Combigan® (timolol/brimonidine)] also exist which minimizes the number of eye drop bottles.

Difficulty Administering Medications. Eye drop delivery aids are available for people who have physical difficulty administering their eye medications. The bottle can be placed in these devices, and the device allows the patient to easily squeeze the bottle in the correct position over the eye. One eye medication, Travatan®, offers an aid which electronically monitors doses and offers reminders when doses are due (Figure 12-1). This aid allows providers to download the information to see how adherent a patient has been since their last visit.

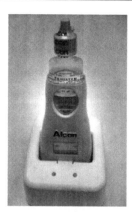

Figure 12-1. The Travatan Dosing Aid®
(Alcon, Ft Worth, TX) reminds patients
when doses are due. It also allows the
eye doctor to download information about
the doses taken and their timing.

Intolerable Side Effects. In general, topical glaucoma eye drops are well-tolerated, especially with the newer generation of medications. Nevertheless, some people can experience untoward side effects. The various medications and the side effects are numerous (see Chapter 7).

High Cost of Medications. In a 3-year review (1998 to 2000) analyzing the medication cost, the following was the cost of glaucoma medication per year (Table 12-1). Some patients are willing to pay more for medications that increase convenience and cause minimal side effects. Others are constrained by the cost, especially when they are taking other medications for systemic diseases.

Table 12-1. Average cost of glaucoma medication per year (1998-2000).	
Cosopt®	$470
Betoptic-S®	$370
Xalatan®	$352
Trusopt®	$288
Alphagan®	$273
Azopt®	$243
Timoptic-XE®	$190
Ocupress®	$183
Generic levobunolol	$138
Optipranolol®	$135
Generic timolol	$133

Figure 12-2. A medication instruction sheet is a helpful reminder to take medications as exactly prescribed (© University of Iowa).

University of Iowa
Department of Ophthalmology and Visual Sciences
GLAUCOMA SERVICE

Name: _____

Date: _____

Action	Medication	Eye	Cap color	Dosing (per day)
☐ Use / Stop	Timolol (XE)	R / L	Yellow	1x / 2x
☐ Use / Stop	Azopt	R / L	Orange	2x / 3x
☐ Use / Stop	Trusopt	R / L	Orange	2x / 3x
☐ Use / Stop	Cosopt	R / L	Blue-White	2x
☐ Use / Stop	Alphagan P	R / L	Purple	2x / 3x
☐ Use / Stop	Xalatan	R / L	White	1x at bedtime
☐ Use / Stop	Travatan	R / L	Aqua	1x at bedtime
☐ Use / Stop	Lumigan	R / L	Aqua	1x at bedtime
☐	_____			
☐	_____			
☐	_____			
☐	_____			
☐	_____			

*This is for your information only - **NOT** a drug prescription.*

Figure 12-2 (continued)

GUIDELINES FOR USING MEDICATIONS

✓ Instill **only one drop** into lower eyelid.

✓ Close eyes gently after each drop for 2 - 5 minutes.

✓ If using more than one drop, wait at least 10 minutes between drops.

✓ Always use drops before ointments.

✓ Place small amount of ointment (size of ½ pea) on eye at bedtime. In the morning, ointment may be cleaned off with clean washcloth.

✓ Once daily medications can be used at any time unless instructed otherwise.

✓ Twice daily medications should be used about 12 hours apart.

✓ Three times per day medications should be taken about 8 hours apart.

✓ Four times per day medication should be taken upon awakening, before bed, and then at two other times, dividing the day as equally as possible.

✓ Please bring all of your eye medications with you for each visit - a list of all other medications you are using would also be helpful.

✓ **DO NOT RUN OUT OF YOUR MEDICATIONS!**

12-B(2). Measures to Improve Adherence to Glaucoma Medications

1) **Understand the Disease and Its Treatment.** Patients are encouraged to ask questions about their diagnosis and understand the rationale behind its treatment. Obtain information on the disease from the prescribing provider, books, and online glaucoma sites (e.g. www.medrounds.org/glaucoma-guide).

2) **Prescribing Least Number of Medications/Doses.** Adherence can be improved by using the least number of medications and least number of doses per day to control glaucoma

3) **Minimize Untoward Side Effects.** Report adverse side effects from eye drops. Understand the expected side effects and identify which ones are not transient. Some medications may cause slight redness upon initial instillation of the drop which improves with time.

4) **Get Written Instructions.** Written instructions are helpful for the patient to recall the exact medical regimen prescribed by the eye doctor (Figure 12-2). Relying only on verbal instructions often leads to mistakes in administration of medications. It is difficult for the patient to remember all verbal instructions when there is so much information given during a clinic visit.

5) **Use Colors to Identify Correct Medications.** It is important to know what medications are prescribed, what they do, and how to correctly identify them. The bottles cap color provides a helpful reminder of what each bottle contains (see Table 7-2).

6) **Practice Administering Medications in the Clinic.** Patients are encouraged to practice administering eye drops under the supervision of their eye doctor or nurse. This allows the eye doctor to

see how well a patient is instilling their medications. It also reassures the patient that their instillation technique is correct.

7) **Time Doses with Scheduled Activities.** Dose eye drops with scheduled activities. Patients can often incorporate their medication in the morning, with meals, and at bedtime. Linking the eye drop with an activity, such as brushing teeth or taking other oral medications, is helpful.

8) **Obtain Help from Family/Caregivers.** Enlisting the help of others may be necessary for those who are unable to comprehend or self-administer eye drops. Family/caregivers' understanding of the disease and its treatment is key to improving adherence to a prescribed drug regimen.

9) **Perform Punctal Occlusion or Eyelid Closure.** It is recommended that patients wait at least 10 minutes between medications to allow better absorption of each medication. If 3 eye drops have been prescribed, there would be 20 minutes of waiting time per dose. For example, if there are 3 medications that need to be taken twice daily each, more than 40 minutes of time is necessary to administer these medications each day. It is easy to see how an increase in the number of medications causes a decrease in adherence. Another method of improving absorption of eye drops is to use punctual occlusion. This maneuver allows the eye medication to absorb more effectively by obstructing the outflow from the eye. It is performed by placing finger pressure over the lower eyelid puncta by the nose (see Chapter 7, Figure 7-6).

10) **Use Eye Drop Delivery Aids If Necessary.** Eye drop delivery aids could be useful in some patients (Figure 12-3). For those with arthritis or severe vision loss, it may be useful.

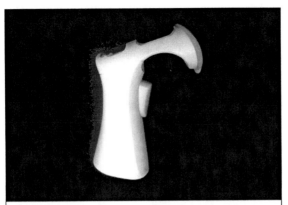

Figure 12-3. An eye drop dispenser for Xalatan®
(Xal-Ease®, Pfizer, NY, NY) can help those who
have difficulty administering Xalatan eye drop.

11) **Checking on Prescription Refills to Determine Adherence Level.** Patients and eye doctors can check on the number of refills within a certain time period. This gives a general estimation to see if the usage seems appropriate.

12) **Generic Drugs and Understanding Available Resources to Decrease Cost.** Generic glaucoma medications are available which helps to defray some of the cost. The Glaucoma Research Foundation (www.glaucoma.org) provides a section on financial aid and programs that assist patients with obtaining their glaucoma medications.

12-C. Low Vision Aids

If glaucoma is undiagnosed or poorly controlled, it may result in varying degrees of visual disability. Once vision loss occurs from glaucoma, it cannot be regained. If the loss is mild, the patient may not experience any limitation in their daily activities. If moderate, there may be some visual impairment. In advanced cases, functional vision can be severely compromised to the point of legal blindness. It is, therefore, important to have periodic scheduled monitoring for glaucoma with good adherence to a prescribed drug regimen. This can minimize the visual decline resulting from glaucoma.

When functional visual disability exists, evaluation by a Vision Rehabilitation Specialist is important. A vision rehabilitation specialist is an eye doctor trained in providing low vision evaluations and presenting devices which may assist patients in their daily activities. The purpose of a Vision Rehabilitation Specialist is to improve individual's activities of daily living (ADLs) so that the disability's effects are minimized. These specialists can assess a person's needs within both home and occupational settings and provide recommendations to improve their level of functioning within these areas. A consultation may provide instruction on the optimal eyeglass prescription (near and far), lighting for various tasks, and an assessment of driving. Various low vision aids may be beneficial, including high prescription reading glasses, filtered lenses, handheld and freestanding magnifiers, talking clocks/books and other appliances, large print materials, electronic reading machines, telescopes, closed circuit televisions/video magnifiers, computer access technology, and devices for Braille. These aids allow patients to optimize their functioning in both home and occupational settings. For example, adequate task lighting and prescription strengths for reading may be evaluated so that reading is easier and more enjoyable. Filtered lenses can help with light sensitivity or problems with glare. Both handheld and freestanding magnifiers are helpful for patients who require increased magnification for better reading. They come in different strengths. Handheld magnifiers have the benefit of being portable but are bothersome for those with hand tremors. Free-standing magnifiers are more useful in these cases but have the disadvantage of not being easily portable. Talking clocks/books and other appliances are also helpful for visually disabled persons. They allow people to rely on their hearing to obtain information. Large print books are helpful for those who need extra magnification for easier reading. These are available in books stores and libraries. Closed circuit TVs/video magnifiers have a camera which magnifies images that are then re-layed to a monitor for viewing. This is useful for reading material such as newspapers or for important activities such as reading bills or signing checks. A vision rehabilitation evaluation aims toward im-proving patients' lifestyles by analyzing their needs and providing the means and methods to meet them.

12-D. Minimizing the Impact of Glaucoma on Lifestyle

A chronic disease requires chronic treatment. The diagnosis of glaucoma often means a lifetime of ophthalmic exams and treatment. Chronic treatment and monitoring should be incorporated into one's life with minimal strain or stress to the patient. One of the major fac-tors affecting how likely a patient will be adherent with medications is the impact of glaucoma treatment on a person's lifestyle. Physi-cally active patients would prefer not to have continual disruptions in their day to administer medications. It is important to minimize the number of medications/doses per day to adequately control glau-coma. The number of prescribed medications increases if glaucoma is uncontrolled with existing medications. Doses per day depend on the type and number of prescribed medications. Once-daily dosed medi-cations help minimize the time requirement for administration.

Incorporating medications into a daily routine helps prevent missed doses. Once a routine is established, there is less of a chance of forgetting medications. Until a routine is established and memorized, it is helpful to have written instructions to follow. This eliminates dosing the incorrect eye or using the wrong number of doses.

When glaucoma surgery is warranted, the type of procedure chosen can be influenced by lifestyle choices. Discuss your activities with your doctor to guide surgical treatment. Input from the patient helps to maximize surgical success.

Cost becomes an issue with using glaucoma medications. The average cost per month can be significant depending on the number of medications used. Generic brands are available for some of the eye drops which can decrease their cost substantially. A prescription health plan and other benefits (e.g., veterans' benefits) also help to defray the cost of these prescription medications. Comparing costs of medications online is another method of finding the most economical alternatives. Using drug delivery aids can prevent wasted doses by effectively delivering the medications to the eye. A discussion with your eye doctor can help devise a plan for the most effective and least costly drug regimen.

Take advantage of low vision aids and existing benefits. Computer monitor settings can be changed to increase font size and appearance of the screen for advanced visual loss. In the United States, a person who has significant vision loss or is legally blind (best corrected vision less than 20/200 or visual field < 20° in the better eye) may qualify for Social Security or Supplemental Security Income (SSI) benefits (www.ssa.gov) or tax benefits (www.irs.gov). Directory assistance and other benefits may be available depending on the state of residence. The Library of Congress (www.loc.gov/nls) also provides free library services for the visually impaired and physically disabled. Veterans may also qualify for benefit through their Veterans Administration (www.va.gov).

12-E. Glaucoma Societies and Organizations

Numerous glaucoma resources are available to patients and eye doctors. The following is a list of the larger national organizations. They each provide links to other organizations and support groups.

The **American Academy of Ophthalmology** (www.aao.org) is the national organization for ophthalmologists. Its membership and resources are extensive. A special Patient section is provided which answers many questions about glaucoma. In addition to providing information on various Eye Health Topics, it contains helpful sections regarding glaucoma.

The **American Glaucoma Society** (www.glaucomaweb.org) is a nationally recognized society whose members are practicing glaucoma specialists. It also provides patients with basic information about glaucoma and its treatment. It is a helpful resource for patients who are looking for a glaucoma specialist in their geographical location.

The **Glaucoma Foundation** (www.glaucomafoundation.org) is a not-for-profit organization which provides patient information about diagnosis and treatment, and provides funding for glaucoma research. Information is presented in an easy to understand format. A PDF of their Patient Guide is available for downloading. Information about support groups for both adult and children is given in associated links.

The **Glaucoma Research Foundation** (www.glaucoma.org) provides funding for glaucoma research. The Foundation provides access to support services and discusses issues regarding financial assistance with glaucoma medications.

Research to Prevent Blindness (www.rpbusa.org) is a non-government organization which provides generous funding for eye research. Basic concepts of glaucoma are discussed and presented. Downloadable articles are also available detailing recent research developments within the field of glaucoma.

Several international groups exist. **The Association of International Glaucoma Societies** (www.globalaigs.org), of which the American Glaucoma Society is a regional member, is an international organization which facilitates collaboration among many glaucoma societies throughout the world. It attempts to distribute and consolidate information regarding the standard practice of glaucoma. **The Association of International Glaucoma Patient Organizations** (www.aigpo.org) arose from The Association of International Glaucoma Societies and provides patients with regional support groups and references regarding patient education.

Finally, this entire book, *A Patient's Guide to Glaucoma*, is available for free online at www.medrounds.org/glaucoma-guide.

References

1. Alward WLM. Glaucoma: *The Requisites in Ophthalmology*. St Louis, Mosby, 2000.

2. Alward, WLM. *Color Atlas of Gonioscopy*, St Louis, Mosby, 1994.

3. Anderson, DR. Collaborative Normal Tension Glaucoma Study. *Curr Opin Ophthalmol*. 2003;14(2):86-90.

4. Ayyala RS, Zurakowski D, Smith JA, et al. A clinical study of the Ahmed glaucoma valve implant in advanced glaucoma. *Ophthalmology*. 1998;105:1968-76.

5. Bartlett JD. Jaanus SD, Fiscella RG, Sharir M, "Ocular Hypotensive Drugs." In Bartlett JD, Jaanus SD, eds. *Clinical Ocular Pharmacology*, ed. 4. Butterworth-Heinemann, Boston, 2001. p.167-218.

6. Bartlett, JD, editor. "Agents for Glaucoma." In *Ophthalmic Drug Facts*. Facts and Comparisons, St. Louis, 2003. p.181-252.

7. Brandt, JD. Corneal Thickness in Glaucoma Screening, Diagnosis, and Management. *Curr Opin Ophthalmol*. 2004; 15(2): 85-9.

8. Busche S, Gramer E. Verbesserung der Augentropfenapplikation und Compliance bei Glaukompatienten. Eine klinische Studie. [Improved eye drop administration and compliance in glaucoma patients. A clinical study]. *Klin Monatsbl Augenheilkd*. 1997;211(4):257-62.

9. Collaborative Normal-Tension Glaucoma Study Group. The effectiveness of intraocular pressure reduction in the treatment of normal-tension glaucoma. *Am J Ophthalmol*. 1998;126(4):498-505.

10. Fingert JH, Anderson, MG. Chapter 144: Glaucoma. In *Emery and Rimoin's Principles and Practice of Medical Genetics*. 5th Ed. Elsevier, Philadelphia, 2007. p.3133-3156.

11. Fingert JH, Stone EM, Sheffield VC, Alward WLM. Myocilin Glaucoma. *Surv Ophthalmol*. 2002;47:547-561,

12. GeneReviews. see tinyurl.com/34eks3 (www.genetests.org/servlet/access?id=8888892&key=3L1fqyZufuJdP& fcn=y&fw=29qT&filename=/reviewsearch/searchdz.html)

13. GeneTests. www.genetests.org

14. Gloster J, Parry DG. Use of photographs for measuring cupping in the optic disc. *Br J Ophthalmol*. 1974;58(10):850-62.

15. Gloster J. Quantitative relationship between cupping of the optic disc and visual field loss in chronic simple glaucoma. *Br J Ophthalmol.* 1978;62(10):665-9.

16. Gloster J. Vertical ovalness of glaucomatous cupping. *Br J Ophthalmol.* 1975;59(12):721-4.

17. Gordon MO, Beiser JA, Brandt JD, Heuer DK, Higginbotham EJ, Johnson CA, Keltner JL, Miller JP, Parrish RK 2nd, Wilson MR, Kass MA. The Ocular Hypertension Treatment Study: baseline factors that predict the onset of primary open-angle glaucoma. *Arch Ophthalmol.* 2002;120(6):714-30.

18. Gurwitz JH, Glynn RJ, Monane M, Everitt DE, Gilden D, Smith N, Avorn J. Treatment for glaucoma: adherence by the elderly. *Am J Public Health.* 1993;83(5):711-6.

19. Hayreh SS. Pathogenesis of cupping of the optic disc. *Br J Ophthalmol.* 1974;58(10):863-76.

20. Hitchings RA, Spaeth GL. The optic disc in glaucoma. I: Classification. *Br J Ophthalmol.* 1976;60(11):778-85.

21. Johnson AT, Alward WLM, Sheffield VC, Stone EM. Chapter 2: Genetics and Glaucoma. In Ritch R, Shield MB, Krupin T, eds. *The Glaucomas.* 2nd Ed. Mosby, Chicago, 1996. p.39-54.

22. Kass MA, Gordon M, Morley RE Jr, Meltzer DW, Goldberg JJ. Compliance with topical timolol treatment. *Am J Ophthalmol.* 1987;103(2):188-93.

23. Klein BE, Moss SE, Magli YL, Klein R, Johnson JC, Roth H. Optic disc cupping as clinically estimated from photographs. *Ophthalmology.* 1987;94(11):1481-3.

24. Kosoko O, Quigley HA, Vitale S, Enger C, Kerrigan L, Tielsch JM. Risk factors for noncompliance with glaucoma follow-up visits in a residents' eye clinic. *Ophthalmology.* 1998;105(11):2105-11.

25. Kwon YH, Caprioli J. Primary Open Angle Glaucoma. In *Duane's Clinical Ophthalmology*, Tasman W, Jaeger EA, eds.; J.B. Lippincott Co., Philadelphia, 1999. Chapter 52:1-30

26. Kwon YH, Kim C, Zimmerman MB, Alward WLM, Hayreh SS. Rate of visual field loss and long-term visual outcome in primary open angle glaucoma. *Am J Ophthalmol.* 2001; 132(1): 47-56.

27. Latina MA, Sibayan SA, Shin DH, et al. Q-switched 532-nm Nd:YAG laser trabeculoplasty (selective laser trabeculoplasty): a multicenter, pilot, clinical study. *Ophthalmology.* 1998;105:2082-8.

28. Lewis RA, Hayreh SS, Phelps CD. Optic disk and visual field correlations in primary open-angle and low-tension glaucoma. *Am J Ophthalmol*. 1983;96(2):148-52.

29. Lloyd MA, Baerveldt G, Heuer DK, et al. Initial clinical experience with the Baerveldt implant in complicated glaucomas. *Ophthalmology*. 1994;101:640-50.

30. Millar, JC, Gabert, BT, Kaufman, PL. Aqueous Humor Dynamics. In *Duane's Clinical Ophthalmology*. W Tasman and EA Jaeger (eds.) Saint Louis: Lippincott Williams & Wilkins, 2005. Chapter 45.

31. Muir KW, Santiago-Turia C, Stinnett SS, Herndon LW, Allingham RR, Challa P, Lee PP. Health literacy and adherence to glaucoma therapy. *Am J Ophthalmol*. 2007;142(2):223-6.

32. Patel SC, Spaeth GL. Compliance in patients prescribed eye drops for glaucoma. *Ophthalmic Surg*. 1995;26(3):233-6.

33. Quigley HA, Green WR. The histology of human glaucoma cupping and optic nerve damage: clinicopathologic correlation in 21 eyes. *Ophthalmology*. 1979;86(10):1803-30.

34. Quigley HA. Early detection of glaucomatous damage. II. Changes in the appearance of the optic disk. *Surv Ophthalmol*. 1985;30(2):111, 117-26.

35. Robin AL, Pollack IP. Argon laser peripheral iridotomies in the treatment of primary angle-closure glaucoma. Long-term follow-up. *Arch Ophthalmol*. 1982;100(6):919-23.

36. Rosman M, Aung T, Ang LP, et al. Chronic angle-closure with glaucomatous damage: long-term clinical course in a North American population and comparison with an Asian population. *Ophthalmology*. 2002;109:2227-31.

37. Sheffield VC, Alward WLM, Stone EM. Chapter 242: The Glaucomas. In Scriver CR, et al, eds. *The Metabolic & Molecular Basis of Inherited Disease*. 8th Ed. MacGraw-Hill, St. Louis, 2001. p.6063-6075.

38. Shingleton BJ, Richter CU, Dharma SK, et al. Long-term efficacy of argon laser trabeculoplasty: a 10-year follow-up study. *Ophthalmology* 1993;100:1324-9.

39. Simmons RB, Montenegro MH, Simmons RJ. "Primary angle-closure glaucoma". In Tasman W ed. *Duane's Clinical Ophthalmology*, Lippincott Williams & Wilkins, Philadelphia, 2005. Chapter 53.

40. Sleath B, Robin AL, Covert D, Byrd JE, Tudor G, Svarstad B. Patient-reported behavior and problems in using glaucoma medications. *Ophthalmology*. 2007;113(3):431-6.

41. Spaeth GL, Hitchings RA, Sivalingam E. The optic disc in glaucoma: pathogenetic correlation of five patterns of cupping in chronic open-angle glaucoma. *Trans Sect Ophthalmol Am Acad Ophthalmol Otolaryngol.* 1976;81(2):217-23.

42. The John and Marcia Carver Non-profit Genetic Testing Laboratory. www.carverlab.org.

43. Vold SD, Riggs WL, Jackimiec J. Cost analysis of glaucoma medications: a 3-year review. *J Glaucoma.* 2002;11(4):354-8.

44. Weiss HS, Shingleton BJ, Goode SM, et al. Argon laser gonioplasty in the treatment of angle-closure glaucoma. *Am J Ophthalmol.* 1992;114:14-8.

45. Wolfs RC, Borger PH, Ramrattan RS, Klaver CC, Hulsman CA, Hofman A, Vingerling JR, Hitchings RA, de Jong PT. Changing views on open-angle glaucoma: definitions and prevalences—The Rotterdam Study. *Invest Ophthalmol Vis Sci.* 2000;41(11):3309-21.

activities of daily living	daily activity a person performs for self-care.
acute angle-closure glaucoma	acute angle-closure glaucoma may present suddenly with pain, nausea, and decreased vision. As its name implies, the drainage angle is closed when examined with a gonioscopy lens.
Ahmed implant	a glaucoma drainage device, a tube shunt with a valve.
alpha-adrenergic agonist, alpha2-agonist	agents that stimulate the adrenergic (sympathetic) nervous system. Stimulation of alpha2 receptors decreases aqueous production at the ciliary body.
amblyopia	lazy eye, a condition in which the visual part of the child's brain does not develop properly due to abnormalities of the eye (for example, glaucoma) or eye alignment (strabismus).
angle-closure glaucoma	glaucoma with closed drainage angle. Can present acutely or chronically.
anterior chamber	the front chamber of the eye.
anti-metabolites	chemotherapeutic drugs often used to increase the success of trabeculectomy surgery.
aphakia	no crystalline lens in the eye due to previous cataract surgery without intraocular lens replacement.
aqueous fluid flow	aqueous fluid is produced by the ciliary body and flows between the iris and lens, through the pupil and to the junction of the iris and the cornea. Aqueous fluid exits the eye through the trabecular meshwork.
aqueous fluid or aqueous humor	clear fluid within the eye.
aqueous suppressants	medications that decrease the production of aqueous fluid.

arcuate visual field defect	an arc-shaped missing area in the field of vision. Glaucoma tends to affect the superior and inferior parts of the optic nerve first, thereby producing inferior and superior arching or arcuate visual field defects respectively.
argon laser trabeculoplasty (ALT)	a common glaucoma laser surgery, performed in an office setting. It uses an argon laser which delivers energy to the trabecular meshwork to increase drainage and lower the intraocular pressure.
axons	nerve fibers.
Baerveldt implant	a glaucoma drainage device. A tube shunt without a valve.
beta-adrenergic blockers or beat-blockers	agents that block the action of the beta adrenergic (sympathetic) nerves. Beta blockers lower intraocular pressure by decreasing the production of aqueous.
bleb	an elevation of conjunctival tissue formed by the aqueous fluid which is being filtered out of the scleral flap (trapdoor) following a trabeculetomy surgery.
bleb-associated endophthalmitis	a bleb infection leading to intraocular infection.
blebitis	infection of a bleb.
bleeding, optic nerve	bleeding or hemorrhage around the optic nerve, common in normal tension glaucoma. It often indicates an ongoing damage to the optic nerve and inadequate control of glaucoma.
blepharospasm	spasm and closure of the eyelids.
buphthalmos	"ox eye," the enlargement of the eye from high pressure in infants with glaucoma.
candidate gene approach	making a list of genes that might cause a disease (such as glaucoma) if their normal function is altered and then testing a large group of unrelated patients for defects in these genes.
carbachol	a cholinergic drug that constrict the pupil and lowers the intraocular pressure.
carbonic anhydrase inhibitors (CAI)	drugs that inhibit the enzyme carbonic anhydrase. CAIs reduce the production of aqueous fluid and thereby lower intraocular pressure.

cataract	cloudy lens which results in decrease in vision. It can also result in thickening and narrowing of the anterior chamber drainage angle.
childhood glaucoma	usually refers to glaucomas that occur very early in life (usually under the age of 3 years). It is also commonly referred to as infantile or congenital glaucoma. When glaucoma occurs between the ages of 4 - 39 years, it is usually referred to as "juvenile" glaucoma.
cholinergic agents	agents that stimulate the cholinergic receptor. Cholinergic stimulation causes increased outflow of aqueous through trabecular meshwork. The pupil also constricts. The topical medications within this class include pilocarpine, echothiophate iodide, and carbachol.
choroidal effusion	fluid accumulation under the choroid space, sometimes seen when the intraocular pressure is very low.
ciliary body	part of the eye between the iris and the retina which produces aqueous fluid.
closed drainage angle	closure of the drainage angle which blocks outflow of fluid from the eye and causes the intraocular pressure to become elevated.
congenital glaucoma, primary	glaucoma occuring in the first 3 years of life without associated ocular or systemic abnormalities.
conjunctiva	a thin tissue that coats the surface of the sclera or eye wall; a thin membrane that covers the eye and lines the inside of the eyelids.
cornea	the transparent structure of the eye in front of the iris and pupil.
corneal edema	abnormal fluid build-up in cornea causing swelling and haziness of the cornea.
cryoprobe	freezing probe, an instrument for applying extreme cold to destroy or ablate a tissue.

cupping	The term "cupping" of the optic nerve describes the appearance of the optic nerve to the examining eye doctor. When the nerve is viewed through the pupil, it has a central cup. The cup is an empty space in the middle of the optic nerve surrounded by optic nerve fibers.
cup-to-disc ratio	a measure to describe the amount of cupping of the optic nerve. The cup-to-disc ratio is often measured to estimate the amount of optic nerve damage. The cup-to-disc ratio of normal subjects is typically around 0.2 to 0.3. Glaucoma subjects have higher cup-to-disc ratios.
cycloablation	destruction of the ciliary body.
cyclocryotherapy	use of a cryoprobe (freezing probe) to freeze and ablate the ciliary body.
cyclophotocoagulation	ablation of the ciliary body using a laser. A procedure to treat a refractive glaucoma which cannot be controlled by medications and other surgeries.
CYP1B1 gene	gene associated with congenital glaucoma.
cystoid macular edema	accumulation of fluid and swelling in the macula of the retina.
cytochrome P450 1B1 (CYP1B1)	a gene associated with congenital glaucoma in patients with a positive family history. Many patients with primary congenital glaucoma (PCG) have the disease due to variations in the CYP1B1 gene.
Descemet's membrane	a layer of cells in the cornea (between the stroma and the endothelium).
diplopia	double vision.
diurnal variation	variations/ fluctuations that occur during the course of a day.
drainage angle	also called "irido-corneal" angle. the angle formed by the iris and cornea where the aqueous fluid drains out of the eye.
drainage tube implant	tube shunt, also known as a seton. Placement of a drainage tube implant that will facilitate the drainage of aqueous fluid and lower the intraocular pressure.

echothiophate iodide	(Phospholine Iodide®); an indirect-acting cholingergic agent which inhibits acetylcholinesterase thereby increasing the outflow of aqueous humor and decreases the intraocular pressure.
epidemiology	study of disease in populations.
epiphora	excessive tearing of the eye.
far-sighted	hyperopia; requires extra effort to focus on near objects.
filtering procedure	a procedure that creates a new passage for aqueous fluid to exit which, in turn, lowers intraocular pressure.
forward bowing of the iris	a key feature of acute angle-closure glaucoma is the abnormal forward position of the iris. Forward bowing of the iris may be observed during an acute angle-closure glaucoma.
fundus camera	a camera designed to take pictures of the retina and optic nerve of the eye.
genetic testing	the scientific analysis of an individual's or family's genetic material (DNA) to determine whether specific genetic mutations exist which result in a particular disease,
glaucoma	a disease of the optic nerve, sometimes associated with high intraocular pressure (IOP) resulting in damage to the optic nerve and vision loss.
glaucoma drainage device (GDD)	also known as tube shunt or seton implant. Tubes attached to a plate, that, when implanted, allow aqueous fluid to drain from the inside to outside of the eye. Ahmed, Krupin, Baerveldt, and Molteno implants are the most common implants available.
glaucoma suspect	those individuals with suspicious findings for glaucoma but without definitive evidence of glaucoma. Glaucoma suspects need to be watched carefully for the development of glaucoma.
glaucoma tube shunt	see glaucoma drainage device (GDD).
glaucomatous optic nerve	progressive cupping of the optic nerve is a typical feature of glaucoma.

Goldmann applanation tonometry	a common technique to measure intraocular pressure (IOP) by placing a prism tip against the cornea and applanating (or flattening) the cornea.
Goldmann contact lens	a specialized lens which is placed on the surface of the cornea for gonioscopy and laser trabeculoplasty.
Goldmann perimeter	a testing device used to test the visual field. The examiner presents the patient with moving test lights of varying size and brightness. Patients indicate that they see a target by pressing a button. The output of the Goldmann perimeter is a manual plotted diagram which is a map of the visual field.
Goldmann, Hans (1899-1991)	a Swiss ophthalmologist who developed and refined many ophthalmic instruments, including the applanation tonometer, slit lamp, bowl perimeter, and gonioprisms/gonio-lens.
gonio-	angle.
gonioplasty	a procedure which uses a gonioscopy lens and a laser to shrink the peripheral iris, which pulls iris away from the trabecular meshwork, opens up the drainage angle, and improves the aqueous outflow. (similar to iridoplasty).
gonioscopy	the use of a specialized lens to examine the drainage angle. The gonioscopy lens is gently held against the cornea to see the trabecular meshwork in the drainage angle
gonioscopy lens	a specialized lens used to examine the trabecular meshwork and iridocorneal angle.
goniotomy	surgery that involves making an incision through the abnormally developed trabecular meshwork to allow greater outflow of the aqueous fluid and thereby, lower the intraocular pressure; commonly performed in congenital glaucoma.
Haab's striae	stretch marks or tears in Descemet's membrane in cornea; commonly seen in congenital glaucoma.

Heidelberg Retina Tomograph	a laser device used to measure the amount of cupping and thickness of the fibers that make up the optic nerve; commonly used as a part of glaucoma care.
hemorrhage	bleeding.
hemorrhage, optic nerve	bleeding around the optic which can be seen in normal tension glaucoma. It often indicates an ongoing damage to the optic nerve and inadequate control of glaucoma.
horizontal raphe	Superior and inferior optic nerve fibers meet at the horizontal midline in the retina referred to as the horizontal raphe,
Humphrey field analyzer	Automated device to measure the peripheral visual field.
hyperopia; hyperopic	far-sighted; requires extra effort to focus on near objects.
hypotony	low intraocular pressure below the physiologic level. Abnormally low intraocular pressure, or hypotony, is one of the complications of trabeculectomy.
infantile glaucoma	see congenital glaucoma.
intraocular pressure (IOP).	a pressure inside the eye that is determined by the production and drainage of fluid (aqueous humor) within the eye. In patients with glaucoma, normal drainage is impaired, which often leads to high IOP.
iridectomy	surgery of the eye to remove part of the iris in order to alleviate pupillary block in angle-closure glaucoma.
irido-corneal angle	the drainage angle of the eye, which is located between the cornea and the iris.
iridoplasty	see gonioplasty
iridotomy	hole in the iris placed to alleviate block in angle-closure glaucoma. See laser peripheral iridotomy
iris	the colored structure in front of the lens which controls the amount of the light that enters the eye. By opening or closing it functions as a diaphragm and regulates the amount of light passing through the pupil
iritis	inflammation of the iris and adjacent structures of the eye

isopters	the circular markings on the Goldmann visual field that represent peripheral vision as tested with various visual targets
juvenile glaucoma	glaucoma that presents between the ages of 4 and 39, and is usually associated with very high intraocular pressure.
juvenile open-angle glaucoma (JOAG)	JOAG patients have very high intraocular pressures that frequently exceed 40 mm Hg in the absence of treatment. In many cases, JOAG runs in families as a dominant trait. See juvenile glaucoma.
Krupin implant	a glaucoma drainage device; a tube shunt with a valve
laser iridotomy contact lens	a specialized contact lens that allows a magnified view of the iris architecture for use in laser peripheral iridotomy
laser peripheral iridotomy (LPI)	a laser procedure that places a hole in the iris to prevent or relieve the pupillary block, thereby opening up the drainage angle.
laser suture lysis	a procedure performed after trabeculectomy in which flap sutures are selectively cut to increase filtration and reduce intraocular pressure.
laser trabeculoplasty	laser energy is delivered to the trabecular meshwork to increase the outflow and reduce intraocular pressure.
lazy eye	a condition in which the visual part of the child's brain does not develop properly due to abnormalities of the eye (for example, glaucoma) or eye alignment (strabismus). see amblyopia.
legal blindness (legally blind)	In the United States, a person is considered to be legally blind if the best corrected visual acuity is 20/200 or worse, or if the widest visual field is 20 degrees or less, in the better eye.
lens, crystalline	focuses images on the retina and is similar to the lens of a camera.

linkage analysis	a method for identifying disease genes that is dependent on the availability of large families with several members that have the disease. DNA is collected from each member of these families and is tested to see which segments of the DNA are always passed down through the family along with the disease. Genes that cause the disease are located within these linked regions of DNA.
low tension glaucoma	see normal tension glaucoma.
low vision aids	devices such as high prescription reading glasses, filtered lenses, handheld and free-standing magnifiers, talking clocks/books and other appliances, large print materials, electronic reading machines, telescopes, closed circuit televisions/video magnifiers, computer access technology, and devices for Braille which may assist low vision patients in their daily activities.
miosis	pupil constriction
mixed mechanism glaucoma	glaucoma in which there is a component of both closed- and open-angle mechanisms contributing to the development.
Molteno implant	a glaucoma drainage device. A tube shunt without a valve
myocilin	mutation in this gene causes juvenile open angle glaucoma and 3-4% of primary open angle glaucoma in adults. Myocilin associated glaucoma is inherited as an autosomal dominant trait. Sometimes called MYOC or TIGR
myopia, myopic	nearsightedness; difficulty in seeing distant objects.
narrow drainage angle	narrowing of the anterior chamber drainage angle. The narrow drainage angle predisposes the patient for angle-closure glaucoma.
nearsightedness	myopia; difficulty in seeing distant objects.
nocturnal variation	fluctuations occurring at night
non-contact applanation tonometry	a technique to measure intraocular pressure by using an air puff to flatten the cornea.

normal tension glaucoma	a significant portion of glaucoma patients do not have elevated intraocular pressure; this subgroup of patients is often referred to as having "normal tension," "normal pressure," or "low tension" glaucoma.
OCT	see optical coherence tomography
ocular hypertension	elevated intraocular pressure beyond normal range.
optic nerve	a nerve that travels from the back surface of the eye to the brain; carries all visual information from the eye to the brain.
optic neuropathy	a general term used for any condition that damages the optic nerve.
optical coherence tomography (OCT)	uses a laser source to scan a cross-sectional picture of the retina and optic nerve. A computer analysis of the cross-sectional picture allows it to measure the thickness of the nerve fiber layer, which correlates with optic nerve damage.
Optineurin (OPTN)	Mutations in this gene are responsible for a significant fraction of normal tension glaucoma with family history.
outflow drugs	medications that facilitate the outflow of aqueous fluid from the eye, and thereby lower the intraocular pressure.
pachymeter	an instrument used to measure corneal thickness
pachymetry	measurement of corneal thickness
pediatric glaucoma, (childhood, infantile, congenital) glaucoma	glaucoma that occurs in infants, usually under the age of three years.
perimeter	a device used to assess peripheral vision.
perimetry	a diagnostic procedure which measures peripheral vision; see perimeter
Perkins tonometer	a hand-held device used to measure the intraocular pressure.
photophobia	sensitivity to light.
pigment dispersion syndrome	a cause of secondary open-angle glaucoma in which iris pigment disperses into the drainage angle blocking aqueous flow thereby elevating intraocular pressure.

pilocarpine	a direct-acting cholinergic medication. It increases the trabecular meshwork aqueous outflow, and thereby lowers the intraocular pressure.
plateau iris configuration	a forward rotation of the ciliary body, which causes narrowing of the drainage angle peripherally.
Posner gonioscopy lens	a specialized lens used to examine the drainage angle.
primary angle-closure glaucoma (PACG)	glaucoma associated with closure of the drainage angle; can present in either acute or chronic form.
primary congenital glaucoma (PCG)	a glaucoma that occurs in the first 3 years of life without associated ocular or systemic abnormalities.
primary open-angle glaucoma (POAG)	glaucoma associated with open drainage angle.
prostaglandin analog	medication to improve the nonconventional outflow (uveoscleral outflow) and lower the intraocular pressure.
pseudoexfoliation syndrome	a syndrome in which white, flaky material is deposited in the drainage angle, increasing the intraocular pressure leading to glaucoma
ptosis	drooping eyelid
punctal occlusion	occluding the tear drainage from the eye by pressing on the tear ducts near the inner lower corner of the eyes with fingers; a method meant to improve absorption of eye drops and to decrease systemic side effects.
pupillary block	can cause angle-closure in which aqueous is trapped behind the iris pushing it forward to obstruct the trabecular meshwork.
Raynaud's phenomenon	can cause cold and numb fingers due to poor peripheral blood circulation.
retina	the tissue of the eye that senses light and functions like the film of a camera
retrobulbar anesthetic	injection of anesthetic behind the eye
Schlemm's canal	a circular channel in the eye that drains aqueous humor from the trabecular meshwork.
sclera	the eye wall; the white part of the eye
scotoma	a blind-spot; a visual field defect

secondary open-angle glaucoma	glaucoma caused by decreased aqueous outflow through the open angle due to blood, inflammatory cells, pigment, and other known causes
selective laser trabeculoplasty (SLT)	a procedure that utilizes a neodynium:YAG laser which targets the trabecular meshwork to increase the outflow and lower the intraocular pressure.
seton implant	see glaucoma drainage device (GDD)
suprachoroidal hemorrhage	intraocular bleeding at the level of the choroid.
surgical iridectomy	see iridectomy
target intraocular pressure	The goal intraocular pressure at which glaucoma is expected to be stable.
TIGR	see myocilin
tonometry	the measurement of intraocular pressure
trabecular meshwork	the drainage structure located in the iridocorneal angle
trabeculectomy	a filtering procedure which creates a small hole in the anterior chamber of the eye to allow drainage of the aqueous fluid toward the outside; a commonly performed glaucoma surgical procedure to lower the intraocular pressure.
trabeculectomy filtering bleb	see bleb
trabeculotomy	a surgery that involves inserting a fine instrument into the Schlemm's canal, and breaking through the trabecular meshwork to increase the aqueous outflow; commonly performed in congenital glaucoma
uveoscleral outflow	non-conventional outflow; provides aqueous outflow through the ciliary body face and iris.
Vision Rehabilitation Specialist	an eye doctor trained in providing low vision evaluations and presenting devices which may assist patients in their daily activities.
visual field	includes both central and peripheral vision. The visual field is measured by a device such as the Humphrey Field Analyzer.
visual field defect	a missing area (scotoma) in the field of vision

Index

D

E

F

G

H

I

J

K

L

M

N

O

T

U

V

Printed in the United States
139420LV00005B/85/P

9 780979 707513